skinny**juices**

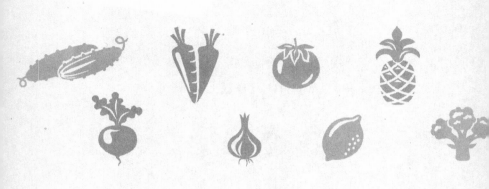

skinny**juices**

101 Juice Recipes
for Detox and Weight Loss

Danielle Omar, MS, RD

Da Capo

LIFE
LONG

A Member of the Perseus Books Group

All rights reserved. No part of this publication may be reproduced, stored in a retrieval system, or transmitted, in any form or by any means, electronic, mechanical, photocopying, recording, or otherwise, without the prior written permission of the publisher. Printed in the United States of America. For information, address Da Capo Press, 44 Farnsworth Street, 3rd Floor, Boston, MA 02210

Set in 11.5-point Adobe Caslon Pro

Library of Congress Cataloging-in-Publication Data is available for this book.

ISBN 978-0-7382-1757-4 (paperback)
ISBN 978-0-7382-1758-1 (e-book)

First Da Capo Press edition 2014

Published by Da Capo Press
A Member of the Perseus Books Group
www.dacapopress.com

Note: The information in this book is true and complete to the best of our knowledge. This book is intended only as an informative guide for those wishing to know more about health issues. In no way is this book intended to replace, countermand, or conflict with the advice given to you by your own physician. The ultimate decision concerning care should be made between you and your doctor. We strongly recommend you follow his or her advice. Information in this book is general and is offered with no guarantees on the part of the author or Da Capo Press. The author and publisher disclaim all liability in connection with the use of this book.

Da Capo Press books are available at special discounts for bulk purchases in the U.S. by corporations, institutions, and other organizations. For more information, please contact the Special Markets Department at the Perseus Books Group, 2300 Chestnut Street, Suite 200, Philadelphia, PA, 19103, or call (800) 810-4145, ext. 5000, or e-mail special.markets@perseusbooks.com.

10 9 8 7 6 5 4 3 2 1

To my mom, who always knew I had it in me.

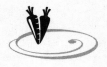

contents

PART THREE
LET'S GET JUICING

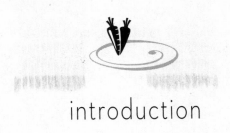

introduction

AS A REGISTERED DIETITIAN, I've seen firsthand the benefits of adding fresh juices to your life. I also know there is a lot of misinformation and debate surrounding juice and juicing. So before we get to the good stuff, let me start off by telling you what I know juicing is *not*.

Juicing is not a diet. It's not the answer to all of your health problems. It is not going to cure you of any disease. Juicing alone is not going to undo the effects of years and years of unhealthy eating habits. So, if you're reading this book in hopes of juicing doing any of those things, you can stop reading now.

Phew! Now that we've gotten that out of the way, let's get busy talking about what juicing *is*. Juicing is a lifestyle. Juicing is transformative. Juice is an infusion of nutrients and phytochemicals that will help heal and nourish your body. Juice is delicious! As part of a clean eating, detox-friendly lifestyle, juicing is all of those things. I know this to be true because I live it and I've witnessed it.

Over the last few years I've led hundreds of people through my Clean Eating Detox. In this twenty-one-day group program, eager participants agree to trade in a diet of highly processed, pro-inflammatory, and toxic foods for one filled with whole foods, very few animal products, and tons of delicious green smoothies and juice. My intention for creating the detox right from the get-go was to inspire people who wanted to make radical dietary and mind-set changes. People who were looking for a way to detox away from their old eating habits while trying out a new way of thinking about food.

My intention for *Skinny Juices: 101 Juice Recipes for Detox and Weight Loss* is the same. More than just a book of juicing recipes for weight loss and detox, I wanted to create a resource—a guidebook for harnessing the delicious power of green juice, clean eating, and living a detox lifestyle.

I want you to change the way you think about food and challenge what you've been told about healthy eating—and juicing. I want you to read this book, start juicing and changing your diet, and have an unforgettable experience. I want you to feel each day how food can affect your mood, energy level, ability to focus, and overall attitude. I also want to show you that living a detox lifestyle each and every day is possible, long after your program is over. And don't worry, if you've experienced the power of juicing already, you'll still find plenty of info here—plus some delicious new recipes to add to your repertoire. I've always believed that the journey to abundant health is so much more than simply removing certain foods from your diet. Of course, removing highly processed foods full of sugar, sodium, and artery-clogging fat is important, but you don't achieve abundant health just by avoiding unhealthy foods. The foods that you *add* to your diet are just as important as the foods you take away. A healthy body is created from the inside out. It happens over time, and with consistent effort. I truly believe it's your everyday eating decisions that will have the most influence on your body and mind in the long run.

In this book I will teach you the ins and outs of juicing. I will also help you design your own personal clean eating detox. You will learn how to change the landscape of your plate to include foods that support your body's own detoxification pathways and help to create wellness from the inside out. Yes, juice plays a large role in this transition, but it doesn't end there. Juicing alone is not the answer—you must also pay closer attention to where your food comes from, how much it's processed, and how it's prepared.

I'm also going to help keep you juicing and eating clean, whole foods long after your detox is over by teaching you the daily practices that encourage a detox lifestyle. You're going to wonder how you can feel completely full and satisfied by eating less!

This book brings together the main philosophies of my Clean Eating Detox program and 101 juice recipes that support weight loss, detoxification, and digestive health.

But that's only part of what you can expect from this book. You can also expect safe and effortless weight loss. Whether it's your last five pounds or your first fifteen, once you start drinking my delicious juices and following the detox protocol, you will see a new "skinny" you come shining through. And the "skinny" you isn't just losing weight on the scale. You're also losing the baggage that comes with eating an unhealthy diet. All the guilt, shame, and regret that's been weighing you down will become a part of the past as you let go of your old ideas about what you should eat and start feeling better than you ever have before!

And if that's not enough, here's what else you're going to learn:

- The science behind juicing

- The difference between juicing and blending

- How to choose a juicer and prepare your kitchen to make juicing and living a detox lifestyle a breeze

- Which fruits and vegetables juice well and which ones do not

- How to juice on a budget and build your juicing menu around the freshest produce

- What to juice when targeting specific nutrients

- How to design your own clean eating detox— employing the same ideas, principles, and practices I use with my own clients

- Tips and strategies for living a detox lifestyle

I hope you use this book as a way to create abundant health and ultimate wellness in your life! I believe it's the perfect place to begin your journey, a delicious place to stay and explore for a while, and a safe place to return to again and again.

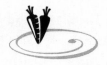

how to use this book

THE BOOK IS ORGANIZED into three sections.

In Part 1 you'll learn of the many benefits of juicing, my philosophy about it, and the scoop on the latest research. You'll also learn how to choose the best juicer for your lifestyle and how to prep your kitchen to make juicing as simple as possible.

In Part 2 you'll learn all about toxins and toxic overload, your body's natural detoxification process, and how juicing is the perfect complement to living a low-toxin, detoxifying lifestyle. You'll learn which fruits, vegetables, herbs, and other foods are the most detox-friendly and how to incorporate them into your everyday life. You'll also learn how to design and implement your own detox and weight loss plan, utilizing clean whole foods and the delicious juice recipes in this book.

In Part 3 we're getting our juice on! Here you'll find 101 amazing juice recipes, organized by their ingredient benefits: cleansing and detox, weight loss, immune defense and antioxidant power, anti-aging, digestive health, and cancer fighting. You'll also discover delicious superfood juice add-ins, plus tips and strategies for juicing while on a budget. You'll even learn which vegetables to juice if you're looking to target specific nutrients.

As an added resource, you'll also find the available nutritional information for every juice recipe, including calories, carbohydrates, sugar, fats, protein, fiber, and key nutrients like iron, vitamin K, vitamin C, and more. This will make your weight loss efforts much easier as you will know exactly how many calories you're consuming with each delicious juice.

So, if you're ready to get started, keep on reading. And get ready to change the way you think about food!

PART
ONE
why juice?

If you're totally new to juicing and want to lose excess weight and detox your body, you are in the right place! I can't wait to teach you about the wonderful health benefits of juicing, the difference between juicing and blending, how to choose a juicer, plus a few easy ways to prep your kitchen to make juicing a cinch. Once you've taken these few preparation steps you will be well on your way to having more abundant energy and vitality than ever before.

Juicing Benefits
and Philosophy

THE NUTRITION WE GET from plants is abundant and amazing. Plants are really the most nutritious foods you can eat. Fruits, vegetables, and greens are rich sources of antioxidant vitamins A, C, and E, and important minerals like iron, potassium, calcium, and magnesium. They're also rich in fiber, which keeps your digestive tract healthy and helps to lower cholesterol.

But vitamins, minerals, and fiber are not all you get from plant-based foods. They also contain thousands of other

What Are Antioxidants?

Antioxidants are substances that protect your cells from the damaging effects of free radicals. Free radicals are molecules produced when your body breaks down food, or by environmental toxins like tobacco smoke, pesticides, and radiation. Free radicals are believed to play a role in the formation of heart disease, Alzheimer's disease, cancer, and many other diseases.

disease-fighting compounds called phytonutrients. Phytonutrients are an important part of a plant's self-defense system. They are compounds inside of plants that provide them with antioxidant protection from the same things we face—ultraviolet light, radiation, toxins, and pollution. They also protect plants against predators and pests.

Phytonutrients are classified by their chemical structure and then grouped into different families. For example, flavonoids and phenols are an important family of antioxidant compounds that have been studied extensively for their beneficial effects on human health. Research has revealed their antiviral, anti-inflammatory, and anticancer properties. You are more familiar with these compounds than you think. Flavonoids are what give blueberries and grapes their blue and purple color. They are what make green tea so good for you and they give garlic its antioxidant punch.

Another group of phytonutrients is the organosulfur compounds, found in garlic and brassica vegetables like broccoli and cauliflower. These powerful chemicals have been shown to support the body's natural ability to detoxify pesticides and other environmental toxins. Curcuminoids are a group of polyphonic compounds that play a vital role in reducing inflammation in the body. Curcumin is the curcuminoid found in turmeric and gives it its yellow color. Curcumin has also been shown to increase glutathione levels in our cells. Glutathione is the body's master antioxidant and plays a major role in detoxification.

Your diet is a powerful player in the fight against many diseases. Consuming foods that are packed with phytonutrients gives your body the ammunition it needs in the fight to stay healthy. The good news is that juicing is one of the easiest ways to get more of these plant nutrients into your diet. Consuming juiced and blended whole fruits and vegetables is the backbone of my detox program and an integral part of living the detox lifestyle.

The Big Debate

Should I juice? Isn't it better to eat your veggies whole? What about the fiber?

I'm asked these questions all the time. As a registered dietitian I've been trained to make dietary recommendations based on scientific evidence. And because of that, I take these questions to heart.

Let's face it, the facts are pretty clear when it comes to fruits and vegetables—the more you can eat, the better! Research shows over and over that fruits and vegetables are excellent sources of the vitamins, minerals, antioxidants, and other nutrients that help reduce chronic disease, increase life span, boost energy and vitality, and promote overall wellness.

Research also tells us that as a nation, we're falling very short when it comes to intake. In fact, a 2009 survey by the Center for Disease Control shows us that just over 30 percent of adults consume fruit two or more times per day, and just 26 percent eat vegetables three or more times per day. There's actually not one US state in which more than 50 percent of its population meets the recommended 4½ cups of fruits and vegetables per day!

In my own nutrition practice I see this all the time. I have clients who can go weeks—that's right, *weeks*—without eating even one fruit or vegetable. And that's not to mention greens. I'm continually amazed at how little greens are consumed. At the very least, a daily juicing habit can help fill in these nutrition gaps by increasing your fruit and vegetable intake, thus making a profound difference in your health.

As for the argument that whole vegetables are "better" for you than juiced, well that's not always the case. Research has shown that juicing can be just as effective as eating the whole food when it comes to reaping the health benefits. The US Department of Agriculture recently analyzed twelve fruits and discovered that 90 percent of the antioxidant activity was actually *in the juice* rather than the fiber.

Let's take a closer look at the most recent findings in support of juicing:

- Juicing increases overall vegetable intake[1] (according to a University of California–Davis study).

- Juicing contributes to weight loss[2] (according to a study by Baylor College of Medicine).

- Compounds specifically found in apple juice slow the progression of heart disease in the same way that red wine and tea do[3] (according to researchers at UC Davis School of Medicine).

- Kale juice lowers cholesterol levels and improves heart disease risk factors[4] (according to research in the *Journal of Biomedical and Environmental Sciences*).

- Carrot juice protects the cardiovascular system by increasing total antioxidant status[5] (according to researchers at Texas A&M University).

- High-risk individuals were 76 percent less likely to develop Alzheimer's disease when drinking fruit and vegetable juices three or more times per week[6] (according to research by Vanderbilt School of Medicine).

- Hesperidin, a compound found in orange juice, significantly reduces blood pressure and other cardiovascular disease risk factors[7] (according to a 2010 study in the *American Journal of Clinical Nutrition*).

- A 2006 study found that the anticancer and cardiovascular benefits of fruits and vegetables may be more attributable to antioxidants than to fiber. Researchers concluded that, in relation to chronic disease reduction, pure fruit and vegetable juices are not nutritionally inferior to whole fruit and vegetables[8] (research published in the *International Journal of Food Sciences and Nutrition*).

So you can see, science is finally catching up to what juicing enthusiasts have known for years—there's powerful nutrition in juice!

But juicing is not only beneficial for lowering disease risk; it's also a great way to get *more* nutrients out of the fruit and vegetables you eat. If you're taking the time and effort to buy and prepare vegetables, you want to get the most from them, right?

Although the majority of Americans eat their vegetables cooked, in some cases cooking veggies decreases the availability of nutrients, especially important antioxidants and other phytonutrients. Further, if you like your veggies *overcooked,* you run the risk of producing byproducts of oxidation, which makes some important nutrients in food difficult to digest and absorb.

When it comes to phytonutrients inside plants, heat can have a negative effect. One reason is that many important nutrients are water soluble, and when vegetables are boiled, these nutrients leach out into the cooking water. Another reason is heat itself. Cooking or reheating foods can diminish their nutrient content because many vitamins and phytonutrients are degraded at higher temperatures.

Heat is especially harmful when it comes to enzymes. For example, myrosinase and allinase are enzymes responsible for converting some of the nutrients inside plants into powerful cancer-fighting compounds. These enzymes are very active in cruciferous and allium vegetables, and are all but destroyed when the vegetables are cooked.

A notable exception to the heat rule is seen with carotenoids, which are powerful plant phytonutrients that help prevent certain forms of cancer and heart disease. Carotenoids are generally more available to the body in cooked vegetables as compared to raw. This occurs mainly because when the vegetable is heated, its cell walls are softened, making it easier to extract nutrients from the inside. Interestingly, this need for heat may be lessened when a vegetable is juiced. A study of women who drank vegetable juice versus eating cooked vegetables showed almost three times more alpha-carotenoids and 50 percent more lutein in their blood than those who ate the same amount of these carotenoids from cooked food. Why? Because during the juicing process you remove most of the plant's cell walls. This liberates many of the phytonutrients, including carotenoids, making them highly absorbable by the body.

Let's look at some other examples:

- Research shows that beet juice is a powerful nitrate-rich antioxidant. Your body converts the nitrates in beet juice into nitric oxide, a compound that enhances blood flow throughout the body and helps lower blood pressure. When beets are cooked, the nitrate content decreases dramatically. Beets also lose over 25 percent of their folate when cooked. By juicing beets you get more of the phytonutrients that help to keep your heart healthy.

- By juicing raw broccoli you help break down its cell walls and release a cancer-fighting enzyme called myrosinase. This potent enzyme helps your liver to detoxify potentially cancer-causing compounds in your body. Cooking broccoli inactivates this enzyme, so even though steaming broccoli is a healthy way to go, you reap only about a third of its natural cancer-preventing abilities.

- Kale and Brussels sprouts are nutrition power-houses, right? Well, when heated they lose over 50 percent of important carotenoids like lutein, beta-cryptoxanthin, and zeaxanthin, as well as 15 percent of their alpha-carotene, beta-carotene, and lycopene content.

Research reveals the pros and cons of eating your veggies cooked. Indeed, there are advantages to eating vegetables both ways. My advice to you is to maximize your nutrient intake by juicing a variety of fruits and vegetables (including

Allium and Cruciferous Vegetables

Allium Family

Chives	Onion
Garlic	Shallot
Leeks	

Cruciferous Vegetables, Brassica Family

Bok choy	Collard greens
Broccoli	Kohlrabi
Brussels sprouts	Mustard greens
Cabbage	Rapini
Cauliflower	Rutabaga
Chinese cabbage	Turnip

Other Cruciferous Vegetables

Arugula (rocket)	Watercress
Radish	

sprouts, which we get into later) and lightly steaming vegetables when cooking them. At my house, we tend to juice fruits and vegetables that don't make it on our plate that often. For example, I'm not a huge fan of cooked carrots or cooked celery, but I don't mind them at all in my juice. I love that I get to reap the cleansing benefits of these not-so-loved veggies without actually having to taste them. And because I can turn any combination of veggies into a juice, I think of my juice as a supplement, similar to taking a daily multivitamin. Even better is that I can tailor my juice to meet my specific needs, based on what I'm not getting in my diet. You can follow this plan, too—maybe you love carrots and celery but hate beets? Whatever your likes or dislikes, you'll find plenty of juice recipes using a wide range of veggies here.

That being said, I think it's important to reiterate that juicing is a lifestyle and not meant to *replace* eating whole fruits and vegetables in your diet. Juicing is best used as a supplement to a diet that already contains ample amounts of fiber from whole fruits and vegetables, nuts, seeds, whole grains, beans, and legumes.

2

Juicing vs. Blending

 BLENDING AND JUICING are both deliciously healthy ways to incorporate more fruits and vegetables into your diet. I both blend and juice often and I encourage you to do the same; that said, there is a difference between juicing and blending, and for the purposes of this book and a way to jump-start a healthier lifestyle, we'll be focusing on juicing. Here's the scoop:

Juicing

Juicing requires the use of a juicer; there are several different types of juicers you can buy that offer different results (we get into that in the next section). What a juicer basically does is extract the liquid part of the fruit or vegetable from the solid part, leaving much of the insoluble fiber (or pulp) behind. This is beneficial for a few reasons. First, the body doesn't have a ton of fiber getting in the way of digestion. This means all the vitamins, minerals, live enzymes, and other plant nutrients in the juice hit your bloodstream almost instantly, giving you a jolt of energy and vitality. This is great for anyone, but especially the people who struggle to eat veggies because they find them hard to digest.

Second, by separating the nutrients from the fiber, you're able to jam-pack an enormous amount of living, vitamin- and mineral-rich goodness into one glass. A typical morning juice for me might include half a cucumber, one apple, one head of romaine lettuce, one fennel bulb, a handful of kale leaves, two carrots, three stalks of celery, ginger, half a lemon, and whatever else I toss in for good measure. Could I eat all of that produce for breakfast? Probably not. But by juicing in the morning, I'm able to get in all of those nutrients before I even start my day, and I'm also rehydrating my body after hours of sleep.

You might be thinking that this lifestyle could become a strain on your grocery budget. I totally understand! What you'll be surprised to learn is that it all evens out. For one thing, you'll be replacing all that processed and packaged food with delicious, organic produce. You'll also find that you're satisfied with less food. This means you won't be stocking up on all those other foods that leave you feeling empty and always looking for more. Plus there are tons of ways to juice on a budget, which I will tackle in Part 3.

You might also be thinking, *What about the fiber? There's no fiber in juice! Isn't fiber good for me?* It sure is! Fiber is important for a healthy digestive tract and plays a vital role in anyone's diet.

Let's take a closer look at fiber.

There are two types of fiber in the foods you eat: insoluble fiber (does not dissolve in water) and soluble fiber (dissolves in water). Both types are indigestible and found in fruits, vegetables, grains, beans, nuts, and seeds.

Both soluble and insoluble fiber acts as a natural laxative; they soften and bulk your stool and keep it moving through your colon. Insoluble fiber absorbs water, promoting regular elimination and preventing constipation. It's also important in helping to absorb and remove toxic substances that have accumulated in the colon over time.

Soluble fiber is soluble in water and has the ability to form a gel. It acts as a probiotic, which feeds the good bacteria in your gut, improving digestion and the health of your GI tract. It also regulates your blood sugar by slowing down digestion and preventing an elevated insulin response after eating. Soluble fiber is a workhorse in the body. It helps to lower cholesterol, reduce blood pressure and inflammation, and decrease your overall risk of getting heart disease. And guess what? You might be surprised to know that juice contains quite a bit of soluble fiber! The fibrous parts of the plant that stay in the juice are called pectins, gums, and mucilages. We know now that most of the fiber removed in the juicing process is the insoluble kind.

Blending

Now that you know how juicing works, let's look at blending. I actually love blending, too, but it's totally different from juicing. For one, no fancy equipment needed; just a regular blender will do and you're ready to go. Next, you're not separating the liquid and fiber from the produce. Instead, you're blending it all up together, usually with some liquid, into a smoothie-like drink. The process of blending makes a smoothie less of a nutrient powerhouse compared to juice, because you're pulling in lots of air when you blend and this increases oxidation. Remember, the more oxidation you have, the more nutrient loss.

Another difference with blending is that by keeping all the fiber intact, you're asking your body to do a lot more work digesting. This slows down how fast the nutrients reach your cells . . . and how you feel after you drink it. That being said, smoothies keep you full! You can make a meal out of your smoothie by blending in nuts and nut butters, seeds, yogurt, protein powder, and many other fun add-ins. This gives your smoothie an altogether different nutrient profile than you get from juice, and why smoothies are often used to replace a meal.

Now before we move on, there's one more thing to consider with both juicing and blending, and that is sugar content. A super-sweet juice or an all-fruit smoothie can cause your blood sugar to spike, which can lead to health problems. When you first start juicing and blending, it may take a while to get used to the taste of your green drink without lots of added fruit. This is totally normal. When juicing, I recommend you work up to using only one fruit for every three to four vegetables and greens. For blending, add no more than one cup (or one whole fruit) per smoothie. This will help balance the natural sugars from fruit and prevent any unwanted side effects.

Equipment Guide

Now that you are aware of the health benefits of juicing, you need to select a juicer and stock your kitchen with the proper tools to make juicing quick and easy.

Choosing a Juicer

There are several different types of juicers on the market, and choosing the right one for your specific needs is important.

Juicers are typically divided into four main types: centrifugal, masticating, twin gear, and hydraulic press. Each machine operates a little differently and has its pros and cons. Generally speaking, the faster the speed (or rpm) of the juicer and the more heat produced, the less the quality and volume of juice you will get. You may be okay with sacrificing a bit of quality for time saved in the kitchen, and that's totally fine. However, if juicing has been recommended as a remedy for healing, I recommend you spend a little more time and money on juicing.

Now, before we get started, let's look at five main questions you should consider when thinking about which type of juicer to buy.

1. What is your juicer budget?

2. Do you want to make and store large batches of juice?

3. What type of produce do you want to juice (fruit, greens, vegetables, sprouts, herbs, wheatgrass, etc.)?

4. How much time do you have in your day for juicing and for cleanup?

5. How much space do you have in your kitchen to store a juicer?

These questions will help guide you in purchasing the right juicer for your individual needs. Once you've thought about these questions, you can begin looking at the different types of juicers to determine which type meets most of your needs.

I have outlined the different types below, along with the pros and cons of each. They are listed in order by price, quality of juice, and juice yield.

Centrifugal Juicers

These are "drink and go" juicers. They're perfect for anyone new to juicing because they're fast, easy to assemble and clean, and fit most any budget. These juicers work by forcing the produce down a chute into a fast spinning disk blade that sits inside a mesh basket. The juice is then pushed through a fine strainer via centrifugal force into an external juice container.

Pros: Easy to assemble and use; wide-mouthed produce chute allows for less prep time chopping; works well with most fruits and nonleafy greens; least expensive; easy to clean, and widely available.

Cons: Higher speed creates a more foamy juice; enzymes and nutrients are oxidized at a much faster rate; not suitable for juicing wheatgrass and leafy greens; produces the least amount of juice, and can leave behind a wet pulp; juice is best consumed immediately.

Masticating Juicers

These juicers may also be known as slow juicers, cold press, single gear, or single auger juicers. They work by grinding the produce through a super slow spinning auger (with no blades) that gently crushes and squeezes the juice from the produce. The process is slow, allowing for less oxidation and nutrient loss as compared with centrifugal juicers.

Pros: Easy to assemble and use; well suited for juicing leafy greens, herbs, and sprouts; some are able to grind nuts and grains; higher juice yield and slower speed results in less oxidative damage and a higher nutrient content; produces less foam and separation compared to centrifugal juicers; can make juice in large batches for storage up to forty-eight hours with minimal nutrient loss.

Cons: Slower speed means more time in the kitchen; more moving parts may take longer to clean; smaller produce chute means more time chopping and prepping produce for juicing; more expensive than centrifugal juicers.

Twin Gear Juicers

These juicers might also be called dual-gear or triturating juicers and are second only to the hydraulic press in terms of quality and juice yield. They work by using two slow-moving spinning gears to squeeze and press the juice out of the produce and many contain magnets inside the gears to prolong nutrient retention. They come in electric and manual hand-crank versions which are designed specifically for juicing wheatgrass.

Pros: Produces an excellent quality juice with high retention of nutrients; can juice most fruits and vegetables, leafy greens, sprouts, herbs and wheatgrass; can grind grains and nuts; can juice in large batches for storage up to forty-eight hours with minimal nutrient loss.

Cons: Slower speed means more time in the kitchen; more moving parts may take longer to clean; more costly than masticating or centrifugal juicers; juices soft fruits like mango and pineapple poorly.

Hydraulic Press Juicers
These juicers are the cream of the crop! They produce the highest yield and highest quality juice. They work by slowly and gently pressing the juice out of the produce, leaving most of the nutrients intact.

Pros: Excellent quality juice due to very little oxidation and nutrient degradation; can be used for most fruits and all vegetables, greens, herbs, and sprouts; can make large batches that can be stored for up to seventy-two hours.

Cons: Slowest to juice; may be very loud; hardest to clean; significant investment; juices wheatgrass poorly.

When making this important initial decision, most people are deciding whether to go for a blade-type, which is faster and less expensive, or a masticating type, which is slower, can be more expensive, and yields a more nutrient-dense juice. The good news is that these recipes will work with whichever juicer you choose.

Once you've narrowed down which *type* of juicer you want, you can start shopping! When comparing the different features for each machine, keep these tips in mind:

Read the Comments. If buying online and someone takes the time to write a review on the machine you're considering, read it! You can learn valuable tips and insights into how the machine works that you won't learn from the manufacturer.

Compare Features. Look for juicers that eject the pulp outside of the machine and not into an internal basket. This will allow for less cleanup time and a higher juice yield. Also look for multiple speed options rather than just an on/off switch. This will allow you to extract the most juice out of your produce.

Wide Mouthed Feeder Tube. Cut your juicing prep time in half by selecting a juicer with a wide feeder tube at the top, allowing larger pieces of fruits and vegetables to fit through.

Know Your Horsepower. A juicer with lower horsepower will need to run at very high speed, or revolutions per minute (rpm). For optimum nutrient-retention, you want a machine with ⅓ to ½ horsepower or a lower rpm.

Less Is More. Make sure the juicer is not too complicated! You want a juicer that's easy to use, doesn't have a lot of parts to assemble, and is easy to clean.

And remember, the least expensive option is not always the best option. When buying appliances over the years, I've opted many times for the cheaper route—only to end up re-buying that same item over and over because it just didn't last. Think of your juicer (and the time you spend using it) as an investment in your health and vitality. I think you'll be pleasantly surprised to see how little you'll spend on over-the-counter medicine and trips to the doctor once you begin living this lifestyle.

Other Useful Kitchen Tools

I absolutely love a good kitchen gadget, especially one that makes my life easier in the kitchen. When it comes to juicing, there are a few must-have kitchen tools that will make prepping and storing your produce a breeze. Check out the Resources section for retailers.

Vegetable Peeler: If not juicing organic produce, I peel the skin off certain fruits and vegetables. Refer to the Dirty Dozen and Clean Fifteen lists on **pages 48 to 50** to check out the good, and the not so good, when it comes to pesticide use on produce.

Veggie Scrub Brush: Even when I'm using organic produce, I like to give my fruits and veggies a little scrub before juicing.

Mason Jars: I use Mason jars for storing and drinking my juice. I especially love the Mason jar drinking lids from Cuppow.

Juicing Bowl or Basket: I keep the produce I use specifically for juicing in a "juicing basket" in my fridge. This cuts down on prep time and gets me in and out of the kitchen faster.

Green Bags: Evert Fresh Green Bags will extend the life of your produce—something everyone can use!

Good Knives: If you haven't invested in a good set of knives, I highly recommend you do so! My chef's knife is my best friend in the kitchen and a partner in living the detox lifestyle. I know choosing a knife set can be overwhelming and expensive. A great all-purpose knife is the Victorinox Forschner 8-inch Chef's Knife. It's highly rated and costs under $25.

Cutting Board: My large cutting board is my other best friend in the kitchen! Wood and bamboo are the best choices. To prevent cross-contamination, make sure to keep your produce board separate from your meat and poultry cutting boards.

Colander/Strainer: A staple for rinsing produce.

Salad Spinner: Also a staple for washing greens. I clean all my leafy greens at the start of the week to make juicing an easy part of my morning routine.

There you have it! Keep in mind that these items are not essential for juicing; they just make your life a little easier and the entire process a bit more enjoyable.

Now that you've chosen a juicer and your kitchen is prepped and stocked . . . you're ready to start juicing! You may want to go straight to Part 3 and get your juice on. If you want to explore a more concrete detox plan, just turn the page.

designing your detox

Detox is all the rage right now—and it can be an intimidating concept. But when I refer to detox, I don't mean a regimented, unpleasant diet. I mean a journey to health and wellness, rooted in nutrient-dense plant foods, tailored to fit your lifestyle. In this part, I'll demystify detox and show you how you can create a plan that's right for you. You'll learn how to eliminate foods that are making you feel bad and get on track to overall health and vitality. And of course, I'll teach you how to incorporate fresh juices into your day so even if you're not quite ready for a "full" detox, you can still reap the benefits of these life-giving drinks!

3

Why Detox?
Benefits and Philosophy

I'VE ALWAYS CONSIDERED the change of seasons as a time for personal reflection and renewal. It seems that as the weather changes, my body changes with it. Not only do I wear different clothes, I also eat, feel, and move differently. I especially enjoy the transition to eating season-appropriate foods. In the summer I love to feast on watermelon and in the fall I can't wait for my first bite of a Honeycrisp apple! I also like to take stock of what's going on in my life overall: my health, fitness, relationships, and work.

- Am I moving my body every day?

- Am I doing work that feels good to me?

- Am I carving out enough time for myself, as well as my family and friends?

- Am I learning new things and being creative?

- Am I taking on too much?

- Am I feeling burdened or resentful about my obligations?

- Do I feel weighed down?

And of course I must look at my food choices, as they are usually reflective of what's going on in my life.

- Have I been making health-supportive decisions about what I eat?

- Am I eating on the run or relying on convenience foods?

- Am I taking the time to be present at the family dinner table?

- Am I modeling good habits for my daughter?

Taking this time to analyze how I've been eating allows me to mindfully pull back from the foods that make me feel bad and return to the foods that make me feel good. It's sort of like a journey home.

I know in your life you have your own personal health concerns, and that's why I want to help you to design your own personal detox. Because in order to get the most from it, your cleansing ritual should work with the rhythm of your life and meet your personal needs. It hardly ever works to be bound by someone else's dogmatic principles, and detoxing is so much more than going on a juice fast or another diet. It's about becoming aware of how you've been eating, how you've been treating yourself, and how you're feeling as a result.

But remember, changes that are really comfortable for me could be way too intense for you. That's why it's super important to honor your own likes and dislikes and be realistic about what's possible for you. If you are someone who lives off processed foods, just removing these foods from your diet is a kind of detox. If you eat the same foods over and over, just infusing your cells with nutrient-rich juice can be a huge boost to your immune system. This helps you detox because it increases the effectiveness of your own natural detox pathways. Everyone is coming to detox from a different place, and it's important to respect that.

So what does it feel like to detox? What are the health benefits? What can you expect?

Let's take a closer look.

Philosophy and Benefits

There are many reasons that you may choose to detox. As you go through the process on your own, you'll find that the reasons you started with may be completely different from the benefits you experience at the end. Participants in my Clean Eating Detox program experience a wide array of results.

Some of the potential benefits you may experience are:

- Allergy relief

- Blood sugar balance

- Getting off medications

- Hormonal balance

- Improved digestion

- Improved lab values

- Increased energy and mental clarity

- Increased feelings of well-being

- Lower blood pressure

- Radiant skin

- Relief from aches and pains

- Tissue regeneration

- Weight loss

Another great benefit of my Clean Eating Detox is the awareness you gain about how certain foods make you feel— physically and emotionally. Your palate will change and you'll have a whole new understanding of how your body responds to the food you put in it! You also gain a whole new level of food confidence. I talk about food confidence a lot on my blog (www.foodconfidence.com) and with my private clients. Having food confidence means you're no longer victimized by food. Eating doesn't cause you pain, stress, guilt, or shame. You know what foods make you feel good and what foods make you feel bad and you're able to tackle any food situation with grace, purpose, and a sense of control. And if you do make a "bad" food decision down the road, you'll be so tuned in to your body's response to it that getting right back on track is a breeze.

There are many types of detox programs out there. My program is a food- and juice-based detox. It is grounded in the belief that you can prevent disease, lose weight, and feel fantastic, simply from the amazing power of real whole foods and juice.

The primary mechanism of my detox program is to decrease inflammation and support the liver's natural detoxification process for eliminating toxins. This includes providing the necessary nutrients to your colon, skin, lymphatic system, lungs, kidneys, and bladder. Along with your liver, these other organ systems are essential in the elimination of toxins.

What Causes Inflammation?

Inflammation is a natural response by the body's immune system. It's how the body protects and heals itself—without which we would be in a lot of trouble! There are two types of inflammation in the body, acute and chronic. It's not the short-term, or acute, inflammation that we are trying to reduce during detox. Acute inflammation is a healthy body response that indicates healing is underway.

What we are concerned with is the ongoing, or chronic, inflammation often triggered by an immune system that is way out of balance. Chronic inflammation can be triggered in several ways and differs from person to person. It can be triggered by the body's failure to eliminate what was causing acute inflammation; it can be an autoimmune response, where the immune system attacks your healthy tissue, mistaking it for a harmful pathogen; or it can be due to a chronic, persistent immune system irritant. The more we are exposed to things that compromise our immune system, the more chances that we'll have a chronic level of inflammation in our bodies. These immune system irritants include foods we are allergic or sensitive to, viruses, pathogenic bacteria and parasites, as well as obesity, pollution, alcohol, smoking, fried foods, sugar, lack of nutrients (due to a poor diet), chronic infections, drugs (such as painkillers or antibiotics) lack of sleep, and chronic stress. Chronic inflammation can go on for years and years without your noticing or feeling anything, until eventually it causes disease.

My aim is to help you put things back into balance. We will begin to reverse the effects of a diet that has been running too low on vital nutrients like vitamins, minerals, and fiber and much too high on toxic foods, refined sugar, and unhealthy fats. We will also remove the foods that cause chronic inflammation, particularly those you may be sensitive or even allergic to, and not even know it.

It's these critical dietary factors, along with too little exercise, not enough sleep, and chronic stress that are throwing your immune system into overdrive and causing chronic inflammation in your body. Once you start supplementing your diet with delicious detoxifying juices and clean, whole foods, you will start to rid your body of the toxicity that leads to inflammation.

What Are Toxins and Where Do They Come From?

Toxic substances are all around us, disrupting the proper functioning of our bodies. They're in our food and in the environment. Environmental toxins are like chemical freeloaders that grab a ride into our homes on the products we buy and use every day. I'm talking about items like your dishwashing soap, shampoo, body lotion, deodorant, cleaning supplies, and cosmetics. Environmental toxins are also the product of the industrial industry. Dioxins used in the bleaching of paper pulp and the manufacturing of some herbicides and pesticides have been linked to reproductive and developmental problems, damage to the immune system, hormone disruption, and even cancer.

Toxins are also in the water we drink. Current estimates suggest there are over 2,100 known chemical toxins in tap water. To make matters worse, many of them are potential carcinogens. In 2011, the Environmental Working Group (EWG) looked at municipal water systems across the United States. In their analysis they found chemical pollutants called trihalomethanes in every single water system they tested. These chemicals are formed when chlorine, which is used as a disinfectant, interacts with farm runoff or sewage. These toxic trihalomethanes can build up in our bodies and have been linked to bladder cancer, colon and rectal cancer, birth defects, low birth weight, and miscarriage.

And let's not forget about the toxins in our food supply. Each year we consume about fourteen pounds of food additives. This includes colorings, preservatives, flavorings, emulsifiers, humectants, and antimicrobials, just to name a few.

The average person is exposed to over 100 synthetic chemicals every single day. This makes sense since there are over 80,000 chemicals regularly used in pesticides, herbicides, processed foods, and drugs. If you're thinking to yourself, *"Oh, that's not me, I'm so careful about what I buy and eat,"* you might want to look closer at the facts. In today's world, you really can't be careful enough. If you live on the beautiful planet Earth, chemical toxins are inside your body, and your natural detox systems work hard every day to process them. Look at the perfluorinated chemicals used to make nonstick cookware. These perfluorochemicals are so widespread that 99 percent of Americans have them in their body.

This constant influx of toxins not only negatively impacts your health, but it impacts your waistline as well. Researchers are now finding connections between these everyday chemicals and the epidemic of obesity. Most of us don't consider the connection between toxins and weight gain, but the connection is quite real. Emerging research shows that early exposure to the natural and synthetic chemicals in our food, tap water, and even the air we breathe may predispose us to weight gain and obesity.

These special toxins are known as "obesogens," and they disrupt your body's normal metabolic, hormonal, and developmental processes. They do this by surreptitiously sabotaging your endocrine system and flipping the switch on hormones that reprogram your cells to become fat cells. They also tell your body to burn less fat and cause you to feel hungry—all the time. There are at least twenty toxic chemicals now confirmed to be obesogens, and you'll find high levels of all of them inside your cells. Of these obesogens, the ones you likely encounter on a daily basis are high-fructose corn syrup (HFCS), bisphenol-A (BPA), and phthalates.

HFCS can be found in most of the sweetened processed foods available today. HFCS has been shown not only to increase insulin resistance in the liver, but it also interferes with a hormone called leptin, which tells your body that you're full. This tricks you into thinking you're hungry when you're not and leads to overeating.

BPA is a known endocrine disruptor, linked to cancer, diabetes, obesity, birth defects, brain development disorders, and miscarriage. A chemical found mostly in plastic bottles and the lining of canned foods, BPA gets into your body when it leaches from plastics, most commonly from exposure to high temperatures or highly acidic foods. Its role in weight gain is due in part because it mimics the hormone estrogen, which at high levels can promote fat storage. And, like many of the other obesogens, BPA has been shown to increase insulin resistance. The government estimates that 93 percent of Americans have BPA in their body!

Phthalates are added to plastics to increase flexibility and resiliency and easily leach out of the plastics, especially when exposed to heat. The EPA estimates that more than 470 million pounds of phthalates are produced each year. Studies show that phthalates, like BPA, have some level of estrogenic activity and may also alter thyroid hormone levels.

Many pesticides and herbicides are obesogens as well, as are the steroids and antibiotics given to farm animals. Obesogens are in your nonstick cookware (think Teflon) along with grease-proof food wrappers, microwavable popcorn bags, and waterproof materials. You'll find them in PVC plastics like pipes and vinyl flooring and in your cosmetics, perfumes, and lotions. Obesogens also occur naturally in soy.

Pharmaceutical drugs are also associated with weight gain. In fact, many of the most common medications prescribed today can cause weight gain, including antidepressants, anti-inflammatories, and some high blood pressure medications. Birth control pills have long been associated with weight gain in many women. Even a commonly prescribed diabetes drug specifically used to improve insulin sensitivity has a known side effect of weight gain!

I see the reality of this in my nutrition practice. People come to me after gaining ten, twenty, or even forty pounds of extra weight as a side effect of just a single medication. So one problem may get fixed, but they end up spending months, if not years, trying to take the excess weight off.

These chemical toxins cause weight gain in large part because they can lead to insulin resistance. Insulin is a hormone that allows your cells to use up the sugar you consume. If your cells become "resistant" to insulin, your body is unable to use food as energy. This not only leads to your storing more fat, but it can cause fatigue and increase cravings for carbohydrates.

To make matters worse, in addition to the toxins that come into our bodies from food, water, and the environment, we make toxins ourselves. Free radicals are reactive molecules that occur naturally in the body, but can get out of control and become toxic, especially in the face of a persistent toxic overload.

Reducing your exposure to these toxic chemicals can ease the burden on your body's natural detoxification system and in the process may help you lose weight and prevent future weight gain.

So How Does the Body Deal with All These Toxins?

Our bodies have an extraordinary internal detoxification system. Detox occurs all of the time as a normal body process. Our livers are the first line of defense.

Your liver is responsible for chemically breaking down everything that enters your body. This includes not only the toxic chemicals you come into contact with, but everything you consume—your morning cup of coffee, all your meals, the water you drink, even your supplements and medications.

It's the job of the liver to manage what gets into your bloodstream and how it gets in. It allows for absorption of the nutrients you need and transforms toxic substances into safer compounds that you can eliminate.

Your colon plays an integral part in detoxification. It is a main route of elimination for toxins and waste. An unhealthy colon can mean toxins and other chemicals are not being excreted efficiently. Chronic constipation, for example, can cause toxic substances stored in the feces to be reabsorbed into your bloodstream.

The kidneys are also extremely important in the detox process. They are responsible for filtering toxins from your bloodstream and eliminating them through your urine. Each day, your kidneys remove excess waste and water from about 200 quarts of blood.

With over 80,000 chemicals in use, our body's detoxification system is exposed every single day to over 100 toxins—few of which have been tested for their long-term impact on our health. We also must contend with internal toxins like bacteria, fungus, mold, yeast, and parasites that build up in our bodies over time.

With all of these toxins entering our bodies every single day, isn't it easy to see that our livera are overloaded and overworked? When the liver is overburdened, it loses its ability to detoxify efficiently. When this happens, all the toxins you come in contact with need a place to go. They need a place to hang out, and they'll pretty much set up shop anywhere. They find isolation in your cells, in the fluid between your cells; inside your organs, joints, and fat tissue (they love it in there); in the walls of your intestines; and inside your brain and lungs.

The problem is that once they are stored in this way they're not very easy to eliminate. Over time, the lack of elimination causes the body to become toxic and acidic. When this happens, you start to get sick. The toxic buildup causes a cascade of potentially serious health effects. That's why clean eating and periodic cleansing are so important.

Our bodies are fighting an uphill battle when it comes to toxins. Think about the fact that we're exposed to more environmental toxins in one day than our ancestors were in their entire lifetime!

What are some of the symptoms of toxic overload and inflammation?

- Anxiety

- Bad breath

- Bloating, gas, constipation, and diarrhea

- Canker sores

- Depression

- Difficulty concentrating

- Excess weight or difficulty losing weight

- Fatigue

- Fertility problems

- Fluid retention

- Food cravings

- Frequent colds

- Headaches

- Heartburn

- Insulin resistance

- Joint pain and stiffness

- Metabolic syndrome

- Muscle aches

- Postnasal drip

- Puffy eyes and dark circles

- Sinus congestion

- Skin rashes, hives, and acne

- Sleep problems

- Impaired thyroid function

But even with all of the evidence surrounding toxic buildup and its effects on our health, there's still ongoing debate about the need for periodic detoxing. In fact, you're likely not going to learn much about toxic overload from your doctor. Why? Because many doctors (and even some nutritionists) are still of the very conventional (and unrealistic) belief that the liver can do all of this detox work just fine. Yes, despite the mounting data on the impact that a pro-inflammatory diet has on our health, there are still those in the medical field who say: *You don't need to cleanse. The liver will do this all on its own, regardless of your diet and lifestyle.*

But we know this is just not the case. The level of toxic exposure and pro-inflammatory substances that we encounter today is so much more than the body can handle. If you don't believe me, just look around you. It's evidenced by the fact that we in the United States are the sickest, fattest, and most toxic people in the world.

But you *can* do something about it! You can begin to reverse the unwanted effects of chronic inflammation and toxic overload in your diet and environment by taking the time for a periodic cleanup. By doing this you will not only improve your body's ability to absorb nutrients and eliminate waste, but you will decrease inflammation, increase energy, and release unwanted weight . . . and that's just for starters! If you stay with the detox lifestyle by continuing to juice and eat clean, if you avoid foods that you are sensitive to, and limit your exposure to toxic chemicals, you can expect to experience these amazing results as well:

- Abundant energy

- Better digestion and elimination

- Continued weight loss (if needed)

- Deeper sleep

- Fewer seasonal allergies

- Fewer symptoms of chronic illness

- Increase in concentration and mental clarity

- Less congestion

- Less fluid retention

- Less joint pain

- Radiant skin

By going through the process of detoxing periodically and changing your lifestyle, you will begin to reduce your body's toxic load. You will start to see a decrease in the damaging effects of free radicals, and you will amp up your body's natural defenses with powerful antioxidants you obtain from juicing and clean eating.

The Power of Juice

I know you are ready to get started. Hopefully you've gotten your kitchen prepped, purchased a juicer, and have been experimenting with the delicious juice recipes in this book.

Your daily juice is an important part of your detox program. Not only is it cleansing and detoxifying, but it will also help balance the pH level in your tissues, heal and nourish your gut, and strengthen your immune system.

If you're feeling anxious about getting started, remember this: *You already know what your current diet can do for you.* Are you overweight? Do you not sleep well? Do you have low energy or digestive problems? Do you suffer from

What Is Clean Eating?

Clean eating is a lifestyle. It's a way of eating that includes mostly organic, fresh whole foods that have been minimally processed. It also means eating in a way that minimizes exposure to genetically modified organisms (GMOs), toxic chemical pesticides and fertilizers, as well as artificial flavors, sweeteners, colors, and preservatives. A clean diet consists mainly of fresh fruits and vegetables, whole grains, beans and legumes, and animal products that have been raised in a humane manner, free from synthetic hormones and antibiotics.

chronic body aches and pains? If so, this is your chance to change all that. This is your opportunity to learn what a new way of eating can do for your health and how you feel every day!

In addition to drinking an abundant amount of delicious juice, you're also going to change the way you think about food, how food tastes, your eating habits, and your food cravings. You'll also notice softer, clearer skin, more energy, and increased feelings of well-being. And if you're not sure what any of that means, you'll figure it out soon enough!

Everyone will go about this detox in their own way. You may follow the rules "to a T," or you might pull from it just the things that appeal to you—and that's perfectly okay. For most people, adhering 100 percent to the guidelines is not

What Is pH?

When we talk about pH, we're referring to the acidity level in the body. Our bodies don't like too much acidity, as it's a major cause of inflammation and aging, but going overboard on the alkaline end is not good for us either. In general, we want our bodies to run slightly alkaline, with a pH of between 7.35 and 7.45. The food we eat doesn't directly affect our blood pH; however, the foods we eat can affect how hard our body works to maintain optimal pH. An acid-forming food is one that creates a lower, or more acidic pH. Fruits and vegetables are high in potassium salts, which are a natural pH buffer. When you eat a diet that's high in acidic foods (for example, one that is very high in meat and dairy) and low in alkaline foods (like fruit and vegetables), your kidneys have to work hard to keep your pH in the normal range. It does this, in part, by telling your bones to release calcium and magnesium to reestablish alkalinity. Over time, the body's response to a very high acid diet can deplete your bone minerals and may contribute to osteoporosis.

required to reap the wonderful benefits. You can listen to your body and ease into and out of it, as needed. The choice is yours—this is your personal journey!

As I mentioned, inflammation is a main cause of disease and obesity so we want to limit these inflammatory foods as much as possible. This is why you'll start your detox by removing from your diet some of the main causes of inflammation in the body—highly processed foods, gluten, dairy products, refined sugars, and alcohol. You'll replace these foods with tons of fruit, vegetables, greens, and superfoods that provide your kidneys, liver, and digestive system a chance to do some cleanup. It's best to limit the work of the body during this time, so providing it with as many healing and anti-inflammatory foods as possible is the main goal. Once given the opportunity, these foods will get busy right away, helping to boost and optimize your body's natural detoxification ability.

Remember, your body is constantly giving you an indicator of how your diet is affecting you. Your energy level, mental focus, hair, nails, skin, elimination, and mood can tell you a lot . . . if you're paying attention. Observe these things during your detox and you'll learn a tremendous amount about how certain foods affect you.

During your detox, try to let go of any worries that you're not getting what you need. Don't stress about protein grams or whether you're getting too much or too little of this or that nutrient. Eat an abundant amount of anti-inflammatory, detox-friendly foods and don't allow yourself to feel too hungry or too full during the day. Observe how you feel each day by journaling during the program. Use this as your guide in determining how the program is working for you. And remember, this is a gentle detox program designed to jumpstart your journey to amazing health. The allowed foods may seem restrictive compared to what you're used to eating, but after a few days you will adjust to (and love!) your new routine. Remember also that a big part of this program is about changing behaviors. Get comfortable with the idea that you will be eating, thinking, and behaving differently while on the detox.

Finally, if you're not ready or not interested in doing a full detox program, that's fine too—you can benefit from juicing by incorporating any of the juices into your daily routine. You can either choose by particular concern, from basic cleansing to weight loss to supporting digestive health, or go ahead and choose by ingredients—you can't go wrong!

Let's start designing your detox.

4

Your Daily Detox Plan

The first thing you'll need to decide is how long you want to detox. I recommend a minimum of seven days to experience real changes in the way you feel. For most people a period of fourteen to twenty-one days works well. That might sound like a long time, but keep in mind you'll be eating plenty of solid foods, too. Your main focus during this time is to infuse your body with hydrating and alkalizing juices, plus an abundant amount of fruits, vegetables, greens, and other anti-inflammatory and digestive-friendly foods.

Stocking Your Detox-Friendly Pantry

Once you've decided how long you want to detox, you're ready to stock your pantry. There are specific groups of foods that will support your detox and those that will interfere with and even undermine the process.

As you've probably figured out by now, fruits, vegetables, and greens are the foundation of your detox diet and are definitely detox-friendly. When choosing fruits and vegetables, it's best to go with organic options as much as possible. I know that organic produce is not always available or affordable, but it's highly worth it when you think about your toxic load. If buying organic produce is not always an option, focus on the produce that contains the highest pesticide residue and make sure those items are organic. Use the list below published by the Environmental Working Group as a guide for choosing when to go organic and when it's okay to choose conventionally grown produce. And remember, if organics are either out of your budget or not available to you, it's okay—eating conventionally grown produce is still much better than not eating fruits and vegetables at all.

The Dirty Dozen

Here is a list of produce that should be purchased organically whenever possible:

1. Apples

2. Strawberries

3. Grapes

4. Celery

5. Peaches

6. Spinach

7. Bell peppers

8. Nectarines

9. Cucumbers

10. Potatoes

11. Cherry tomatoes

12. Hot peppers

The Clean Fifteen

Produce that is safe to buy conventional:

1. Mushrooms

2. Sweet potatoes

3. Cantaloupe

4. Grapefruit

5. Kiwi

6. Eggplant

7. Asparagus

8. Mangoes

9. Papayas

10. Sweet peas

11. Cabbage

12. Avocados

13. Pineapple

14. Onions

15. Corn

In addition to fresh juice and an abundance of fruits, vegetables, and greens, **the following foods are your detox-friendly staples:**

- Fresh herbs like cilantro, basil, parsley, and dill plus spices like curry, turmeric, cinnamon, and chili powder

- Sprouts like alfalfa, lentil, quinoa, mung bean, broccoli, clover, mustard seed, and radish

- Gluten-free grains like brown rice, wild rice, quinoa, millet, amaranth, rice noodles, and gluten-free oats

- Beans and legumes (dried are preferred, but BPA-free canned and boxed beans are fine, too) like lentils, black-eyed peas, white and red kidney beans, black beans, garbanzo beans, butter beans, and pinto beans

- Raw or dry-roasted unsalted nuts and seeds like almonds, walnuts, pine nuts, and hazelnuts along with hemp, chia, sunflower, pumpkin, and ground flax seeds (store in the freezer to keep fresh)

- Organic, nondairy, and unsweetened nut milks like hemp, almond, hazelnut, walnut, and coconut

- Organic whole soybeans and fermented soy products like tempeh, miso, and natto

- Organic, pastured or hormone/additive-free eggs, chicken, and turkey

- Fresh or water-packed, wild coldwater fish like wild salmon, cod, sardines, trout, halibut, and mackerel

- Healthy cooking oils like extra-virgin olive oil, coconut oil, and grapeseed oil

What to Avoid While Detoxing

Just as there are foods that support your detox, there are foods that will impede the process. Following are the groups of foods that I recommend you avoid during detox, mainly because they are common allergens, pro-inflammatory, and acid forming.

Refined Sugar

Sugar is probably the most important food to avoid during your detox. Not only does it promote inflammation in the body, it also raises insulin levels, depresses the immune system, and increases hunger. Sugar can also be downright addictive for some people. This is why the only sugar I recommend consuming during detox is the natural kind . . . what you get from delicious whole fruit! Detoxing is a great opportunity to retrain your palate to enjoy the natural sweetness in foods, without the need for added sugars. This means no sweetened sodas, sports drinks, and other bottled beverages, including diet drinks and any form of artificial sweetener (like Sucralose, Aspartame, etc.).

You can practice getting used to the taste of less sugar while juicing by experimenting mainly with the recipes that contain only one fruit and lots of vegetables. Eventually you will learn to appreciate the natural sweetness you get from carrots, beets, broccoli, fennel, and other vegetables.

Gluten

Gluten is a protein found in wheat and related grains like barley, rye, spelt, kamut, and sometimes oats (if they aren't labeled gluten-free). Sensitivities and allergies to this protein are on the rise, possibly from the overconsumption of wheat in the American diet. Wheat is the major dietary source of gluten and it could be leaving you with an inflamed gut, mostly due to the way it is processed. Commercial bakeries use hybridized wheat grains and chemical leaveners to mass-produce the presliced bread you find on the grocery shelf. Unfortunately, the use of these grains may be a driver for intestinal inflammation in the GI tract.

The most serious form of gluten intolerance is an autoimmune digestive disorder called celiac disease that affects 1 in 133 Americans. Gluten sensitivity, a much more common condition, is estimated to affect one-third of the US population and is a major cause of inflammation and gut irritation. Since the main goal of our detox is to decrease inflammation and heal the gut, removing gluten from your diet during detox is an effective way to find out if you're sensitive to it.

As you may know, white and whole wheat flour is made from wheat. In addition to bread and pasta, other foods that contain wheat and/or white flour are boxed cereals, granola, pizza, pretzels, croissants, bagels, cakes, wraps, rolls, biscuits, pies, pastries, battered or bread-crumbed foods, boxed foods, and many other processed foods. Read the ingredients on your food labels during detox!

Dairy

Dairy can be pro-inflammatory and hard to digest. In fact, 60–75 percent of the world's population is unable to digest cow's milk and other dairy products due to lactose intolerance. Milk can also affect your blood sugar, causing an insulin spike that may rival white bread. Dairy has been shown to aggravate irritable bowel syndrome, contribute to sinus problems and ear infections, and cause chronic constipation. It's best to let your body have a rest from dairy while you detox.

Processed Soy

Whole soy foods can be a part of your detox, as they are a good source of quality protein and other plant compounds that help promote good health. Fermented soy foods like miso, natto, and tempeh are the best soy choices because they are easier to digest and add needed nutrients and natural probiotics to your diet. Tofu and soy milk are not in this category and should be consumed in moderation. Many of the soy foods you buy these days are made from GMO soy as well, so it's best to go organic, when possible.

You definitely want to avoid highly processed soy during detox and after. This means stay away from the processed fake meats and burgers, which contain soy protein concentrates and textured vegetable protein, or TVP. Strong chemicals are used to make TVP, and the process leaves behind the fiber and health-promoting nutrients found in the original soybean. Also, the spray method used for drying soy forms nitrates, which can be harmful to your heart, so stick to clean soy choices.

Coffee, Caffeine, and Alcohol

Many of us are addicted to the stimulant rush we get from coffee, soda, and other caffeinated beverages. A main problem I see with coffee is that it's often used to cover up a more serious problem—not enough sleep. Use your detox as a way to get back in touch with your body's natural sleep and wake cycles and get out of the habit of using caffeine to burn the candle at both ends!

In the same way caffeine is a bad habit, that nightly glass of wine (or two) can also interrupt your natural sleep cycles, as well as promote insulin resistance and increased body fat.

Unhealthy Fats

The type of fat you consume can make a big difference in your overall health. Inflammatory polyunsaturated vegetable oils that we limit during detox include corn, soybean, cotton-seed, safflower, sunflower, and canola. Saturated fats to steer clear from are those found in high-fat dairy products, fatty cuts of red meat and pork, as well as processed meats like deli meats, sausages, and bacon. Stick with healthy fats like coconut oil and extra-virgin olive oil.

That's it! Please don't be discouraged; you don't have to remove all of these foods forever. But you do need to give yourself long enough to allow your body to heal, and for you to really notice a difference in how you feel without them.

Phases of Detox

My detox consists of three distinct phases: pre-detox preparation, healing and restoring, and transition.

Phase 1: Pre-Detox Preparation

This pre-detox phase lasts five to seven days and prepares the body for cleansing. The length of preparation really depends on to what extent you need it. If your diet is pretty clean to start (i.e., you don't eat a lot of sugar and refined foods or drink coffee/soda) then just a few days are fine. If you're coming into the detox from a standard American diet, then you may want to give yourself the whole week to prepare.

During this phase you will begin to eliminate sugar, caffeine and/or coffee, and alcohol from your diet. You will begin to incorporate juice once per day—or more, if you like. During this time you will likely feel some of the effects of removing these foods from your diet so be prepared for a few days of headaches. I suggest slowly weaning off the caffeine by a little each day to minimize the unpleasant side effects.

You can also prepare your kitchen for detox by removing non-detox foods and securing the tools and supplies you will use during detox. Of course you will need to invest in a juicer and you many also want to look at purchasing a high-speed blender for smoothies. You can use the detox-friendly food list to create a meal plan and get your pantry stocked for the coming week. Start reviewing the Detox Tips and Strategies and the Daily Detox To-Do list **(see page 60)**. Create a schedule for your self-care. It's best to create a daily routine right from the start so the detox protocol integrates easily with your life. I also recommend setting an intention for your detox during this time. This is pretty simple: Decide before you begin what you would like to achieve as a result of the process and keep this in mind throughout your detox.

Phase 2: Healing and Restoring

Phase 2 is the foundation of your detox and is the longest phase. In this phase you have completely altered your diet to include only the detox-friendly foods and juice. You are avoiding most animal proteins except for cage-free eggs, organic chicken, and coldwater fish and you are staying away from gluten, dairy, and processed or packaged foods. You are consuming juice two or more times each day. You are healing and restoring your body by eating a variety of vegetables, greens, juice, and green smoothies.

This phase can last from seven to twenty-one days, depending on the length you choose for your detox. You may also choose to eliminate animal products entirely during this phase, or just for a few days. Many of my detoxers use this time to experiment with a vegan lifestyle by taking two full weeks in this phase, with the second week being completely meat free.

Phase 3: Transition

During this phase you will start to add back the foods you eliminated during the detox, specifically gluten and dairy products. This phase lasts roughly seven days and is important for identifying any allergies or sensitivities you may have to the foods you eliminated, mainly gluten and dairy.

You should add dairy and gluten back into your diet on different days, and be sure to keep track of any symptoms you encounter while eating these foods. I recommend consuming two servings per day of each food, for two consecutive days. After two days, go back to phase 2 detox eating for a day, then you can introduce another food the following day.

Let's look at how that would look for gluten. To add gluten back into your diet you could have bread with your lunch and pasta for dinner. Do this for two days, keeping track of how you feel afterwards and noting any undesirable effects. Some signs to look out for are bloating, gas, bowel changes, fatigue, or headache. Notice *anything* that feels different from how you felt during detox. Then take a day off and go back to phase 2 eating. Follow the same process for dairy, adding in two servings per day for two days, again noting any reactions you may have.

Once this is complete, you can start to add back to your diet the other foods you eliminated during detox (caffeine, sugars, alcohol, etc.). You can choose to follow the same process as above, eating the food being tested twice per day for two days, noting any undesirable effects, or you can gradually add these foods back in, over time.

You may discover that certain foods leave you feeling really good and full of energy, while others cause fatigue, bloating, or even pain. These are valuable messages coming from your body and you definitely want to listen! It makes no sense to regularly consume foods that are irritating to your immune system or that trigger inflammation in your body.

Learning how to live a detox lifestyle will help you maintain the wonderful feeling you had during detox!

Your Detox Strategies

Having guided hundreds of people through my Clean Eating Detox program, I've got a few tricks up my sleeve for enhancing the process and ensuring a great experience.

Here are a few tried-and-true tips and strategies for success:

- Plan your meals over the course of the detox period using a meal planner to get organized; use my sample detox days on **pages 64 to 66** as a guide.

- Space your meals three to four hours apart and don't let yourself get too hungry.

- Schedule snacks midmorning and late afternoon to ward off hunger between meals.

- Minimize over-the-counter medications and avoid reaching for Tylenol or Advil at the onset of aches and pains (but continue taking prescription medications).

- Schedule at least one massage during the course of your detox.

Promoting the release and elimination of stored toxins is a main focus of our detox. Proper elimination and good circulation are very important to your success! The following daily to-do's will help facilitate the process.

Your Daily Detox To-Do List

- Upon rising, consume 6 ounces of warm water with the juice from half a lemon and consider taking a probiotic (see sidebar).

- Consume two servings (8 to 12 ounces equals one serving) of freshly made juice each day, once in the morning and once midday.

- In addition to your juice, drink plenty of clean water. Aim for eight to ten glasses of filtered water each day.

- Keep your bowels moving! If you're not eliminating daily and easily, try a mix of 2 tablespoons ground flaxseed with 8 ounces of cold water before bed.

- Stop eating 3 hours before bedtime.

- Get 8 hours of sleep at night.

- Use a food log daily to record your progress and note how you're feeling during your detox.

- Consciously chew your food. This will aid in digestion, decrease gas, and help assimilate nutrients.

Probiotics—The Good Bugs!

The term "probiotic" literally means "pro life"—and that's exactly what these little bugs are: living bacteria that live inside our bodies and help us maintain optimal health and wellness. Our bodies are made up of ten times more bacterial cells than human cells, and our GI tract is home to over 500 species of them! But these "good bacteria" and other microbes live throughout our entire body, not just in our digestive tract. There are actually 100 known benefits to taking probiotics, among them are a strengthened immune system and a healthy gut. When probiotics are properly balanced and in abundant amounts in your body, it's a lot harder for "bad" bacteria to take over and make you sick. Recent studies show that the type of bacteria in our gut can even determine how easily we gain and lose weight. When choosing a probiotic, aim for 18 to 25 billion cells per dose.

- Take a warm Epsom salt bath (add 2 cups to your bath water) several times per week.

- Dry skin brushing two to three times each week, before you shower (see sidebar).

- Get a good sweat going at least three times a week; go for a sauna, steam, or do hot yoga.

Dry skin brushing is a natural, safe, at-home method for stimulating circulation, removing dead cells, and unclogging your pores. By increasing circulation, you can improve the tone and smoothness of your skin. Dry skin brushing also stimulates the lymphatic system, which can help eliminate toxins from the body. To start skin brushing, purchase a natural bristle brush (these can be found online or at most food stores or pharmacies). Start from your ankles, gently brushing your skin in long strokes towards your heart. Slowly move up your body to your legs, stomach and shoulders, using light but firm strokes. Make long, sweeping strokes on your arms and sides, but use circular strokes for your underarms, wrists, and ankles. Be sure to cover the whole body, but skip your face and breasts.

Side Effects and Weight Loss: What to Expect

Once you've removed the inflammatory and toxic foods from your diet and given your body a rest from the standard American diet, you may start to feel some side effects.

Your body will immediately start getting to work ridding itself of the toxins that have been driven deep into your fat stores and other tissues over the years. Those old toxins will get stirred up and begin to circulate in your blood stream.

As they travel through your bloodstream on their way out of your body for elimination, it can cause some pain in the form of headaches, joint pain, cold- or flu-like symptoms, and fatigue.

If you were a heavy user of caffeine and sugar prior to detox, you may also feel some withdrawal symptoms in the form of headaches.

Although these side effects are unpleasant, know that they last for only three to five days! Try to remember that you're not getting sick, but that you're actually getting better, as your body begins to remove toxic substances from your tissues. So when you start to feel these symptoms, don't give up! Your body is working very hard to clean itself and it needs time to do this important detoxification work. Just take it easy during this time, enjoy some self-care, and know that you are soon going to feel amazing! Use this time to allow the delicious power of juice to aid in the body's ability to detox and cleanse.

Releasing weight is a common side effect of detoxing. Not because you're starving yourself or eating like a bird, but because you're eating less and feeling more satisfied! Also, your body responds to a reduction in toxic load by releasing weight. When you remove toxic and inflammatory foods from your diet and replace them with liver-supporting, nutrient-rich foods, you create an environment conducive to weight loss. When you remove the major causes of bloat, gas, and constipation from your diet, you allow your digestive system to function at its best, eliminating waste quickly and efficiently. The side effect of this is a flatter abdomen (no more gas and bloating) increased energy, and a revved-up metabolism. Detoxing allows you to lose weight naturally without deprivation or dieting!

Sample Detox Days

To help you to plan your detox, below are samples of how I instruct my clients to prepare for and eat during each phase.

Phase 1—Pre-Detox Preparation

To get ready for detox, drink 6 ounces of warm water with lemon in the morning. If you drink coffee, you'll want to start cutting back on that and switch to a substitute such as Dandy Blend (see Resources) or tea. If you're accustomed to desserts, begin to eliminate these. Take a look at your pantry and clear it of any non-detox foods. Incorporate two juices per day into your schedule. You'll also want to meal plan for the week ahead and stock up your fridge.

Phase 2—Healing and Restoring

Upon Rising: 6 ounces warm water with lemon
Morning Juice: *Green Machine (page 127)*
Breakfast: Scrambled eggs with baby spinach and sliced avocado
AM Snack: *Tropical Greens (page 99)*

Lunch: Big green salad with chopped vegetables, avocado slices, cooked lentils, and sunflower or pumpkin seeds, tossed with homemade dressing made with apple cider vinegar, miso paste, and olive oil

PM Snack: O_2 Builder *(page 124)*

Dinner: Organic wild-caught salmon with quinoa and broccoli, tossed with same dressing from lunch

After Dinner: Herbal tea + probiotic

Phase 2—Healing and Restoring
(Vegetarian/Vegan Option)

Upon Rising: 6 ounces warm water with lemon

Morning Juice: *Green Machine (page 127)*

Breakfast: The Detox Kitchen's Cereal Swag (see Resources) with unsweetened coconut or almond milk

AM Snack: *Tropical Greens (page 99)*

Lunch: Black bean lettuce cups with carrot ginger soup

PM Snack: O_2 Builder *(page 124)*

Dinner: Harvest chili bowl with kale salad

After Dinner: Herbal tea + probiotic

Phase 3—Transition

During phase 3 you'll want to slowly add back the foods you wish to reintroduce to your diet. I have my clients do this over the course of seven to fourteen days, and we keep tabs on how they feel with each new addition. To bring dairy back in, you might add Greek yogurt for breakfast. For gluten, you might have cereal or a slice of sprouted bread with peanut butter for breakfast. For added sugar, you could have a piece of dark chocolate at night and use honey in your tea. The key here is to do this very slowly and stretch it out over several weeks, so you can become familiar with what types of foods cause you digestive stress. This will provide you with important information about how you should eat going forward.

Living the Detox Lifestyle

You've completed your detox. You've taken the time to learn which foods make you feel good and which do not. You've invested in a juicer and made juicing a part of your daily routine. You experienced the increase in energy and vitality you get from juicing and eating clean. You have a sense of empowerment because you know how to feed yourself in a way that supports your long-term health.

Now is not the time back down. You've got a clean slate; let's keep it that way, shall we?

How we continue to live and eat after detox is just as important as detoxing itself. Yes, periodic cleansing is a great practice, but it's not enough to prevent inflammation and decrease our overall toxic load for the long term. Don't get me wrong, detoxification is going to happen. Your body's ability to mobilize and eliminate toxins is an automatic process; it will continue despite the constant barrage of inflammatory foods and chemical toxins coming its way. But the decisions you make about how you eat and live going forward are going to be the difference between abundant health and chronic disease. It's that simple. Detox alone is not the answer. You must continue to replenish the body's antioxidant, vitamin, and mineral reserves, and you do this by continuing to juice daily and by living a detox lifestyle.

A detox lifestyle will allow the continual replenishment of your liver and other detoxification organs with the nutrients they need to keep your toxic burden low. It will supply your immune system the phytonutrients it requires to keep you from getting sick. It will keep your internal antioxidant systems running efficiently, and it will help to minimize your exposure to new toxins.

The following lifestyle choices will help you keep your body's toxic burden low for the long haul:

- Use only natural, toxin-free cleaners to clean your home, or make your own.

- Avoid spraying pesticides or herbicides inside your home or on your property (especially if you have animals that go in and out of your house).

- Remove your shoes when entering your home so as not to track in toxic chemicals and pesticides.

- Read labels carefully and use only natural, toxin-free soaps, shampoos, deodorants, and styling products. Look for hair products that do not contain alcohol, sodium lauryl sulfate, paraben, phthalate or other petrochemicals. Avoid hair spray, perfumes and other skin or hair care products that use synthetic fragrances.

- Use low-toxin makeup and skin creams (avoid products with phthalates, parabens, propylene glycol, alcohols, and fragrances).

- Avoid plastic bottles and containers with the recycling codes 3 (contains phthalates), 6, or 7 (contains BPA) on the bottom. These are most likely to leach plastics into the food or beverage that they contain.

- Do not drink from plastic water bottles; invest in a glass or BPA/phthalate-free bottle instead.

- Consider a water filter to limit intake of bacteria and chemicals.

- Do not microwave your food in plastic containers or plastic wrap.

- Do not wash plastic containers in the dishwasher or under very high heat.

- Choose fresh, whole, and organic foods whenever possible. Avoid highly processed foods and limit prepackaged foods. If you are a meat eater, switch to organic, grass-fed, and free-range meats.

- Minimize consumption of mercury-containing fish and shellfish (large tuna, swordfish, shark, king mackerel, tilefish). Also limit intake of PCBs from farmed salmon and fish caught downstream from wastewater.

- Substitute meat frequently with vegetarian protein sources like beans and legumes, quinoa, peas, nuts, leafy greens, and fermented soy products.

- Choose organic dairy products when possible and experiment with unsweetened nondairy milks like almond, hemp, and coconut.

- Reduce your high-fructose sugar intake and avoid artificial sweeteners. When you do use a sweetener, consider natural sweeteners like dates, real maple syrup, agave, stevia, and coconut sugar.

- Exercise regularly.

- Drink alcohol in moderation.

PART
THREE
let's get juicing

Whether you're putting together your own detox plan, look-ing to add more juices to your diet, or hoping to address a specific health concern, this next section will give you the keys: juicing ingredients, how-to, and 101 delicious recipes.

Chapter 5 gives you the skinny on ingredients and tips for juicing on a budget, the juicing process, and working with the recipes. Then it's on to the recipes! If you're looking for detox support, check out Chapter 6. The recipes in Chapter 7 are all designed to help support healthy weight loss. In Chapter 8 you will boost your immune system with juice. Want glowing skin? Look no further than Chapter 9. If you need a little digestive help, Chapter 10 is great for that. And Chapter 11 provides high-powered, anti-cancer recipes.

5

Ingredients and Juicing Tips

JUICING IS A GREAT WAY to enjoy fruits and vegetables that in the past you may not have liked. Oftentimes the juice from vegetables tastes very different from the veggie in its whole form. As I mentioned before, celery and carrots are a great example of this, neither of which I particularly like on their own, but I love to include in my juice. You might find that you dislike beets or Swiss chard, but juicing them brings a whole new flavor sensation to your palate. Another benefit of juicing is that you can quickly and easily juice and consume four to five vegetables at once, which would normally take quite a while to individually prepare and eat. I love to experiment with different flavor combinations that I wouldn't normally eat together if they were cooked. This chapter gives you all the info you need on ingredients, as well as tips for quick and easy juicing.

Juice Upgrades and Superfoods

Fresh herbs like cilantro, basil, parsley, and mint are juice staples. They increase the flavor of your juice and are an important part of detox. Spices like cinnamon and turmeric add superfood power to your juice and are easy to incorporate. I use herbs and spices frequently in my juice recipes and I encourage you to play around with different flavors and varieties as often as you can!

There are so many ways to take your juice to the next level. Superfoods are a great way to get more nutrients (and taste) into your juice. You can garnish your juice with a sprinkle of cayenne for a spicy kick, chopped avocado for texture, cinnamon for added sweetness, or cacao nibs for a dessert-like feel. Let's look at a few upgrades and add-ins that you'll find throughout my recipes.

Aloe Vera. Aloe juice is very soothing to the lining of the intestines and can have a positive effect on digestion. It helps to balance acid and alkaline levels in the stomach and ease gut irritation. It's also a potent antifungal, antiviral, and anti-inflammatory that can help with yeast overgrowth by

What Are Superfoods?

Superfoods are foods that are rich in the nutrients shown to improve your health and prevent disease. They include antioxidants, anti-inflammatories, and cancer fighters. They can be super high in fiber or other phytonutrients like carotenoids or flavonoids. Superfoods include blueberries, nuts, super seeds (such as chia and hemp), and green leafy vegetables like kale, collard greens, and Swiss chard. Cruciferous vegetables like Brussels sprouts, cauliflower, cabbage, and broccoli are also considered superfoods, as are fatty fish like salmon, mackerel, and sardines and some wild mushrooms. Raw cacao is a superfood, too, along with spices like turmeric and cinnamon.

promoting the growth of good bacteria and increasing regularity. Aloe vera gel is best blended rather than juiced. I recommend buying the juice from your health food store and adding it to your recipes. Be sure to look for juice that does not have any added sugar or other ingredients.

Avocado. I love to finish my savory smoothies with chopped avocado. This nutrient-dense superfood is a source of anti-aging vitamin E plus healthy fats that will help keep you full. Avocado also helps the body produce natural glutathione, a compound that is necessary for the liver to cleanse harmful toxins.

Cayenne Pepper. Along with bell peppers, jalapeños, chile peppers, and paprika, cayenne pepper is part of the Capsicum family. Its active ingredient is capsaicin, which is responsible for the boost in metabolism you get from cayenne. It also has cancer-protective, anti-inflammatory, and pain-relieving effects. Use cayenne with some caution, add only a pinch to your juice. Eating too much capsaicin can cause stomach irritation and pain. Also, capsaicin can interact with certain medications (stomach-acid reducers and blood thinners), so consult your doctor before using cayenne pepper if you take these medications.

Chlorella. Chlorella is a single-cell, freshwater algae that is rich in protein, vitamins, and many minerals. It is a true superfood and a natural chelator, known for its ability to bind and remove mercury that's accumulated in the intestines.

Cinnamon. Cinnamon is a natural sweetener and is a great add-in to juice. It helps stabilize blood sugar levels and is a natural antibacterial and anti-inflammatory. It also has a natural warming effect to help you sweat out those toxins!

Cacao Nibs. Cacao beans are the seed of the South American evergreen cacao tree and are used to make cocoa, chocolate, and cocoa butter. Cacao in its raw, unprocessed form is a source of iron, fiber, calcium, zinc, and potassium. Raw cacao nibs are also a good source of antioxidant flavonoids that promote cardiovascular health and protect against toxins.

Chia Seeds. Chia seeds are a wonderful plant source of healthy omega-3 fatty acids, protein, and calcium. They promote a healthy digestive tract, reduce inflammation, and can lower blood pressure. Chia seeds are also high in fiber—they can absorb ten times their weight in water so they're great for adding fiber to your juice!

Coconut. Adding coconut to your juice will not only remind you of the beach, it will also give your metabolism a boost! Coconut contains a special kind of fat called medium-chain fatty acids (or MCTs) that the body digests easily and converts to energy. It's also a great anti-bacterial, anti-viral, and anti-fungal. You can add coconut to your juice in various ways—try mixing in a tablespoon of melted coconut oil, sprinkle on some unsweetened shredded coconut, or stir in a few ounces of unsweetened coconut water.

Flax Seeds. Ground flax is high in omega-3 fatty acids and fiber and is commonly used in detox to help flush toxins from your body. It's also been shown to reduce cholesterol levels and decrease blood pressure. Stir a tablespoon of flax into your juice to create your own delicious high-fiber drink! (Note: flax seeds should always be ground before using.)

Ginger. I find it hard to juice without ginger! It's my favorite add-in, and I love the spice and warmth it brings to the juice. Ginger is a fantastic anti-inflammatory and antioxidant and is widely known for its anti-nausea effects. Recent research also suggests that the antioxidants in ginger may slow the growth of cancer cells.

Kelp Powder. Kelp and other sea vegetables are some of the most nutritionally dense foods on earth. They are an abundant source of natural minerals and chlorophyll. Kelp is a deep green sea vegetable that is very blood purifying and acts as a powerful detoxifier and chelator. Stir a spoonful of kelp powder into your juice for added minerals.

Matcha Tea Powder. Matcha tea is a special variety of green tea in which the whole, powdered leaf is consumed rather than the infusion of the leaves. It is a great source of antioxidants and phytochemicals that have been shown to improve cholesterol, increase metabolism, and lower overall cancer risk. Matcha is also rich in a polyphenol called EGCG (epigallocatechin gallate), which is a potent and health-protective antioxidant. Add matcha powder to any juice for an added boost of antioxidants.

Reishi Mushroom. Reishi mushroom extract is known for its powerful immunity boosting and anti-inflammatory properties. Reishi provides natural energy and can help with daytime fatigue (without affecting your sleep). I use reishi extract in the liquid form and add a few drops to my sweeter juices, as the fruit masks the woody flavor of the reishi well.

Sprouts. Sprouts are an amazing, nutrient-dense superfood. They are loaded with minerals like zinc, cobalt, phosphorus, potassium, magnesium, and calcium. Broccoli sprouts are especially high in cancer-fighting antioxidants, along with potassium and vitamins A, B, C, and K. When juicing sprouts, I like to roll them up in a romaine lettuce leaf to aid the juicing process. The sprouts best for juicing are alfalfa, clover, mung bean, sunflower, radish, and broccoli. See **pages 84 to 85** for more on sprouts and sprouting.

Spirulina. Spirulina is a micro-algae that is an abundant source of complete plant protein. It is actually one of the most concentrated protein sources on earth and contains more protein than beef! Studies show Spirulina also helps to control blood sugar levels and can help prevent cravings. Add Spirulina powder to any juice.

Turmeric. Turmeric is a liver-loving spice. In addition to its proven anti-cancer benefits, it also helps boost liver detoxification and is a potent anti-inflammatory and antioxidant. The medicinal properties of curcumin, its main health component, have been the subject of thousands of studies to date. You can juice turmeric in its root form or buy it as a powder and add to your juice.

Wheatgrass. Wheatgrass is the sprouted grass of wheat seed. It is rich in antioxidants and amino acids as well as vitamins C, E, K, and B_{12}. It is also a source of calcium, cobalt, germanium, iron, magnesium, phosphorus, potassium, protein, sodium, sulphur, and zinc. Because it is sprouted, wheatgrass does not contain gluten. There are only a few studies to date that have tested the potential health benefits of wheatgrass. Preliminary research suggests that wheatgrass may help ease the symptoms of ulcerative colitis. You can consume wheatgrass either as a powder or by juicing it. Keep in mind that to juice wheatgrass properly, you need a masticating hand-crank juicer (see Resources). Wheatgrass is best consumed alone and you should not exceed 1 to 2 ounces, twice per day.

Juicing on a Budget

Buying fresh, organic produce can get expensive. It's a fact that the most nutritious foods tend to cost a little more. There is a way around it, though—a way that makes the idea of spending a bit more each month on the food you eat a little easier to digest. It starts with your mind-set.

If you shift your mind-set to think of buying fresh produce for juicing (and for eating) as an investment in your long-term health, the cost gets a little easier to swallow. For one, you're investing in your immune system. By doing this, you don't get sick as often. This will save you money on over-the-counter medicines each winter when everyone around you is getting sick and you remain healthy and strong. I can attest to this first hand! I rarely get sick from the common cold and flu bugs that go around my house—and I have a first-grader at home, so I am definitely exposed! In fact, my daughter also benefits from this lifestyle, as she rarely gets sick. This investment in your immune system will save you money and time. No taking off work to go to the doctor, no co-pay, no expensive antibiotics or medications and with all that, less toxins entering your body and no side effects from medication.

In addition to changing your mind-set about the cost of fresh food, there are other tips and strategies I've learned over the last twenty years eating a plant-based diet that will make the lifestyle easier on your wallet.

- Shop smart and stretch your budget as far as you can. If you want to invest $25 in juicing per week, pay attention to when produce goes on sale and build your juice menu around these weekly in-store deals. Look for ways to save by buying larger quantities (in bags or in bulk).

- Check out the Dirty Dozen and Clean Fifteen lists on **pages 48 to 50**; it's a great guide to the produce you really should buy organic, if you are prioritizing and budgeting.

- Streamline your grocery shopping by creating a juice theme or menu each week (even better, create it around what's on sale!). Don't buy extra produce that's not on your juicing list for that week.

- Build your juice menu around high-yield produce. Leafy greens and berries are great, but they produce a lot less juice than cucumbers and romaine. Stick to high-water veggies as your juice base.

- Buy seasonally and locally. In-season, locally grown produce is going to be less expensive than something grown far away and shipped. If oranges aren't in season, don't buy them! If you're not sure, a farmers' market is a great place to find out what's in season right now in your part of the country. Build your juicing theme or meal plan around these foods.

- Switch out in-season or on-sale produce when juicing from a recipe. It really doesn't matter if you use an orange or a pear, your juice will still be delicious and nutritious!

- Grow your own produce! Fresh herbs, zucchini, cucumber, peppers, lettuce, and tomatoes—these are all pretty easy to grow in most backyard gardens.

- Not a green thumb? Learn to sprout. All you need are a few glass jars and some cheesecloth. One inexpensive bag of beans or legumes can provide sprouts for weeks and weeks.

- Find a co-op in your area. Local cooperatives are a great way to get organic produce for less.

- Store your produce properly. Wash and prep your leafy greens, wrap in a damp paper towel and store in a plastic bag or Evert Green Bag—this alone will extend the life of your greens tremendously! Store all other produce in the crisper compartment of your fridge.

- Keep your leftover stalks and stems for juicing. I have a bag in my fridge where I store all my produce "spare parts." Stockpile your asparagus tips, beet greens, celery ends, broccoli stems, carrot peels, pineapple cores, parsley stems, and kale stems for juicing.

Juicing Tips

I've got you covered with 101 healthy and delicious juice recipes, but there are a few tips and tricks that will help make juicing a more enjoyable experience. Below are my best tips for getting the most out of your juicing efforts.

- Collect and place all your juicing ingredients in a bowl near your chopping board to get started. Wash, peel (if needed), and chop your produce first.

- Organic produce is going to be your best choice when juicing, especially if you prefer to keep the peels and skin on. Refer to the chart on **pages 48 to 50** to determine which fruits and vegetables are safe to buy conventional and which are best bought organic. Also, even when buying organic, remember to give your produce a good rinse before juicing.

- Stems and seeds are usually fine to juice, however citrus seeds can be bitter and apple seeds can be toxic. See the list on **pages 90 to 92** for more detailed guidance on what part of your produce is safe to juice and what should be avoided.

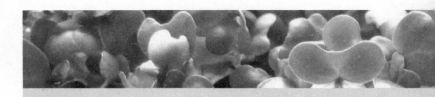

Benefits and Philosophy

What Are Sprouts?

Sprouted seeds are a great addition to your diet. When seeds, nuts, beans and grains are germinated in water, they are transformed into sprouts. Sprouts are good for you because they are nutritional superstars, housing highly digestible energy, live enzymes, bioavailable vitamins, minerals, amino acids, and other phytochemicals. Many seeds turn to sprouts after just a few days sitting on your kitchen countertop! Experiment by sprouting mung bean, alfalfa, lentil, or quinoa seeds to add a delicious array of nutrients into your juice and your meals. For everything sprout-related, visit sproutpeople.org.

Five-Step Guide to Sprouting at Home

Step 1: Choose which seed, nut, whole grain, or legume you want to sprout.

Step 2: Place 2 to 3 tablespoons of your chosen seed into a large Mason jar and cover with water. Place a square of cheesecloth or muslin fabric over the top of the jar and secure with a rubber band. Soak seeds in the water overnight.

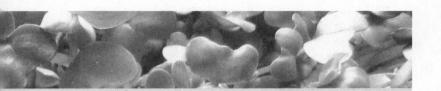

Step 3: In the morning, rinse the seeds a few times through the cheesecloth with fresh cold water. Drain most of the water out of the jar (do not leave the seeds too wet, they need only to be moist). Store the jar upside down in a bowl on the countertop away from direct sunlight. Rinse the seeds twice per day after the morning rinse. I suggest rinsing them once you arrive home from work, and then again before bed. Do this for 2 to 6 days.

Step 4: Once the seeds have sprouted (usually between 2 to 6 days, depending on the seed) remove them from the sprouting jar and eat within a few days.

Step 5: Store uneaten sprouts in a plastic bag in the fridge, making sure they are not damp (run them through a salad spinner) and are well ventilated. A resealable bag left slightly open works great!

Photo of broccoli sprouts by Julie Gibbons

- Save the leftover parts of vegetables that you don't cook and juice them. For example, save the stems from broccoli, the base of cauliflower, kale stems, the core of pineapple, the stems and leaves of beets and fennel, the outer leaves of Brussels sprouts, and the tops and bottoms of bell peppers. I keep a "stem bag" in my fridge and I add to it each day and then juice its contents every few days.

- Fresh is best when it comes to juice! To get the most nutrient bang for your juicing efforts, try to drink your juice within 20 minutes of preparing. If you must store your juice for later, store it in an airtight container in the fridge, leaving very little airspace at the top. Remember, masticating juicers produce less oxidation than centrifugal juicers, so juices made with masticating juicers can be stored for up to forty-eight hours and still maintain nutrient quality. If juice storage is super important to you, invest in a twin gear or triturating-type juicer. These juices can actually be stored for up to seventy-two hours and still retain nutrient quality.

- When juicing greens and fresh herbs, roll them up in a lettuce leaf or wrap the herbs around a celery or carrot stalk. This will make them denser and less likely to spin around in your juicer, so you'll get more liquid out of them.

- The fibers in soft fruits like pineapple and mango can sometimes block the filter of the juicer, so it's best to juice these types of fruit last.

- For the best results, keep the juicer running for about fifteen seconds after the last bit of produce is juiced to allow all of the juice to exit the juicer. There's no specific order in what to juice first, but I tend to juice harder veggies and fruits (beets, carrots, apples) first, and softer fruit like mango and pineapple last so they don't block the filter.

- If you hate the mess of the pulp bin, line it with a bio-degradable bag or a waste bag before juicing. This will save you some cleanup time, and it's an easy way to collect and transfer the pulp if you want to use it in another way, or to separate it from the trash for composting. You can also try stirring a few scoops of it back into your juice for some added fiber!

- Speaking of pulp, before you toss it, rejuice it! I tend to have juicy pulp so I always send it back through the juicer one more time—just to squeeze a few more ounces of juice out!

- For easier cleanup, run some water through your juicer after you're finished juicing, and always rinse and clean your juicer as soon as you've finished using it.

The Pulp

One more reason I don't worry too much about not getting the fiber from my juice is because I repurpose my pulp—and you can, too! You absolutely don't have to toss all of that fiber into the compost or the trash; you can reuse it in a tasty meal or snack.

Below are a few creative ways to make the most out of your pulp:

- Add carrot, kale, beet, celery, or tomato pulp to pasta sauce

- Layer pulp into lasagna

- Mix zucchini, parsnip, or sweet potato pulp into veggie burgers

- Add a scoop of any pulp into your dog's food bowl

- Bake apple, zucchini, or carrot pulp into muffins, loaves, or cakes

- Stir pulp into warm mac and cheese

- When creating your own juice recipes, remember to stick with the proper ratio: one fruit for every three to four vegetables and greens, or aim for 75 percent vegetable and 25 percent fruit!

- I recommend you drink your juice on an empty stomach.

- Make a veggie dip by mixing pulp into cream cheese

- Stir a scoop of pulp into cottage cheese for a snack

- Add savory pulp to soups, stews, or chili

- Mix pulp into lean ground beef for meatloaf or meatballs

- If you have a dehydrator, dehydrate the pulp to make raw crackers

- Add fruit pulp or carrot pulp to pancakes or breads

- Mix sweet potato pulp with mashed potatoes

- Add fruit pulp to homemade frozen popsicles

- Sauté pulp on the stove and serve with a poached or fried egg on top

- Add pulp to smoothies for extra fiber

Still not sure what to do with it? Freeze it until you get inspired!

Recipe Notes and Tips

Fruits, vegetables, greens, and herbs are going to be the foundation of your juice. As I mentioned already, while it might be tempting to juice using more fruit than veggies, it's actually better to juice mostly vegetables, especially if weight loss is your goal. Juice containing too much sugar from fruit can take away from the health benefits of juicing, lessen the effects of detoxification, and prevent weight loss. Most of my recipes use either one or two fruits, so you're going to be fine if you stick with the recipes found here. However, if you're finding it difficult at first, add a little more fruit. It's more important to me that you love juicing, so if fruit is vital to your enjoying your juice, then adjust the recipes accordingly.

Given all the versatility you get with juicing, there are still some parts of fruits and vegetables that you shouldn't juice. It might be due to water content or consistency, or just for safety reasons. Let's take a closer look at which produce makes great juice and which does not!

Can I Juice That?

A common question you'll hear in my house is *"Can I juice that?"* I love experimenting with a different vegetable blend and creating a new favorite juice. For me, most of the produce I eat cooked can also be juiced. This may not be the case in your house, as it really depends on your diet. Most produce that has a high water content can be juiced. I would not juice bananas, avocado, or eggplant, for example.

A good rule of thumb is that if you can eat it cooked, you can probably juice it—with a few notable exceptions.

Seeds and Pits

The seeds in lemons, limes, grapes and some melons may be run through the juicer, but not the large pits from plums, apricots or peaches. Apples should always be cored before juicing as the seeds can be toxic and should not be juiced.

Skin and Peels

If you're not using organic produce, then you should remove the skin and peels to reduce your exposure to pesticide residue. With organic produce you have a little more flexibility, but most fruits and vegetables (especially apples and cucumbers) have tons of nutrition in the peels! Oftentimes it comes down to personal preference.

Juice the following fruits and vegetables with the skin and peel ON:

- Apples

- Beets

- Carrots

- Cucumbers

- Ginger

- Grapes

- Honeydew (skin may be too hard for some juicers)

- Jicama

- Kiwi (you can also peel these)

- Lemon and lime (you can also peel these down to the white pith)

- Mangos
- Nectarines
- Parsnips
- Peaches
- Pears
- Plums
- Sweet potatoes
- Zucchini

Juice these with the peels OFF:

- Cantaloupe
- Grapefruit
- Oranges
- Pineapple
- Pomegranate arils
- Watermelon

And now the very short list of what you just shouldn't juice, whether due to consistency, water content, or safety:

- Avocados
- Bananas

- Carrot greens and rhubarb greens (can be toxic)

- Eggplant

Let's Juice—The Recipes

When using the recipes that follow, refer to the list above to determine what to peel and what not to peel. My recipes assume you are not peeling lemons, limes, or ginger, but feel free to do so if you prefer. Items that should be peeled before juicing are noted. All of the recipes make one to two servings, depending on your appetite!

6

Cleansing and Detoxifying Juices

Kiwi Cleanse

This overall body cleanser and hydrator is the perfect way to get your metabolism revved up to start the day. I just love the sweet and spicy bite of this tropical salsa in a glass!

INGREDIENTS
1 kiwi
½ cup pineapple
2 cucumbers
½ lemon
4 radishes
1 handful cilantro

Juice.

NUTRITIONAL INFORMATION
Calories: 114, *Fat:* 1g, *Saturated Fat:* 0g, *Cholesterol:* 0mg, *Fiber:* 1g, *Protein:* 4g, *Carbohydrate:* 33g, *Sugar:* 18g, *Sodium:* 25mg

SUPER NUTRIENTS
Vitamin C: 194%, *Vitamin K:* 152%

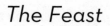

The Feast

Sometimes I like to "juice until dinner." When I do, I make this nutritious juice and sip on it all day long! It keeps me satisfied, hydrated, and well nourished.

INGREDIENTS

1 head romaine lettuce
5 celery stalks
5 kale leaves
3 tomatoes
½ lemon
2 cucumbers
1 red bell pepper
1 garlic clove
1-inch piece ginger
Pinch cayenne pepper

Juice all ingredients except the cayenne pepper. Stir in the cayenne pepper.

NUTRITIONAL INFORMATION
Calories: 220, *Fat:* 4g, *Saturated Fat:* 1g, *Cholesterol:* 0mg, *Fiber:* 2g, *Protein:* 18g, *Carbohydrate:* 54g, *Sugar:* 24g, *Sodium:* 155mg

SUPER NUTRIENTS
Vitamin A: 313%, *Vitamin C:* 405%, *Vitamin K:* 1176%, *Copper:* 262%, *Folate:* 183%, *Iron:* 102%

Spicy Salsa

This spicy juice is both cleansing and nourishing. Garlic contains allicin and selenium, two natural liver cleansers, and cilantro is a powerful chelator and anti-inflammatory.

INGREDIENTS

3 tomatoes
¼ onion
2 garlic cloves
1 red bell pepper
1 handful cilantro
1 lime wedge

Juice tomatoes, onion, garlic cloves, bell pepper, and cilantro. Garnish with lime wedge.

NUTRITIONAL INFORMATION
Calories: 51, *Fat:* 1g, *Saturated Fat:* 0g, *Cholesterol:* 0mg, *Fiber:* 1g, *Protein:* 3g, *Carbohydrate:* 14g, *Sugar:* 8g, Sodium: 24mg

SUPER NUTRIENTS
Vitamin C: 112%, *Vitamin K:* 76%

Tropical Greens

This chlorophyll-rich green juice combines the cleansing power of greens with the tropical taste of pineapple and mint. Add a mini-umbrella to your glass and let it take you back to the beach!

INGREDIENTS
3 kale leaves
3 Swiss chard leaves
1 handful dandelion greens
1 cucumber
2 celery stalks
1 cup pineapple
½ lemon
1 handful mint

Juice.

NUTRITIONAL INFORMATION
Calories: 102, *Fat:* 2g, *Saturated Fat:* 0g, *Cholesterol:* 0mg, *Fiber:* 1g, *Protein:* 8g, *Carbohydrate:* 35g, *Sugar:* 16g, *Sodium:* 297mg

SUPER NUTRIENTS
Vitamin A: 102%, *Vitamin C:* 251%, *Vitamin K:* 1416%, *Copper:* 182%

Clean Green Zinger

This juice is a simple yet powerful way to cleanse your body. The super-hydrating apple and celery are perfectly balanced by the warming spiciness from ginger and the clean taste of cilantro.

INGREDIENTS
1 handful cilantro
4 celery stalks
1 green apple, cored
½ lemon
1-inch piece ginger

Juice.

NUTRITIONAL INFORMATION
Calories: 69, *Fat:* 1g, *Saturated Fat:* 0g, *Cholesterol:* 0mg, *Fiber:* 1g, *Protein:* 2g, *Carbohydrate:* 22g, *Sugar:* 13g, *Sodium:* 53mg

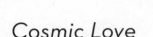

Cosmic Love

This tasty morning juice not only provides the cleansing power of vitamin C and beta-carotene but gives an added boost of vitality from matcha green tea powder.

INGREDIENTS

1 orange
1 red bell pepper
3 carrots
1 lime
1 teaspoon matcha green tea powder

Juice orange, bell pepper, carrots, and lime. Stir in matcha.

NUTRITIONAL INFORMATION

Calories: 87, Fat: 1g, Saturated Fat: 0g, Cholesterol: 0mg, Fiber: 1g, Protein: 3g, Carbohydrate: 27g, Sugar: 15g, Sodium: 77mg

SUPER NUTRIENTS

Vitamin A: 112%, Vitamin C: 179%

Note: Matcha green tea powder not included in analysis

Beet Red

Beets are a detox staple. They are true liver healers with natural anti-aging properties. The compound betaine in beets helps to protect the liver from damage and reduces overall inflammation in the body. This spicy juice is perfect for a crisp autumn morning!

INGREDIENTS
2 beets with greens
5 radishes
1 orange
1-inch piece ginger
1 cucumber

Juice.

NUTRITIONAL INFORMATION
Calories: 107, *Fat:* 1g, *Saturated Fat:* 0g, *Cholesterol:* 0mg, *Fiber:* 1g, *Protein:* 4g, *Carbohydrate:* 41g, *Sugar:* 18g, *Sodium:* 108mg

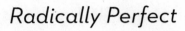

Radically Perfect

High in antioxidants, both radish and grapefruit are very detoxifying. Grapefruit helps boost the liver's production of detox enzymes and contains flavonoids that cause the liver to burn fat, rather than store it. This juice is a natural liver cleanser!

INGREDIENTS
½ grapefruit, peeled
1 small apple, cored
½ lemon
5–6 radishes
1-inch piece ginger
Dash cinnamon

Juice grapefruit, apple, lemon, radishes, and ginger. Sprinkle with cinnamon.

NUTRITIONAL INFORMATION
Calories: 73, *Fat:* 0g, *Saturated Fat:* 0g, *Cholesterol:* 0mg,
Fiber: 1g, *Protein:* 1g, *Carbohydrate:* 24g, *Sugar:* 14g, *Sodium:* 7mg

Weed Whacker

Dandelion greens have great detoxifying and liver-cleansing power. The sweet taste of carrots and apple helps the medicine go down!

INGREDIENTS
1 handful dandelion greens
1 cucumber
3 carrots
1 apple, cored

Juice.

NUTRITIONAL INFORMATION
Calories: 107, Fat: 1g, Saturated Fat: 0g, Cholesterol: 0mg, Fiber: 1g, Protein: 3g, Carbohydrate: 26g, Sugar: 16g, Sodium: 93mg

SUPER NUTRIENTS
Vitamin A: 110%, Vitamin K: 169%

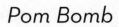

Pom Bomb

I love adding texture and fiber to my juice. Pomegranate arils are antioxidant superstars and add great dimension to this simple juice.

INGREDIENTS
1 handful kale leaves
1 apple, cored
1-inch piece ginger
1 handful mint
1 handful pomegranate arils

Juice kale, apple, ginger, and mint. Stir in pomegranate arils.

NUTRITIONAL INFORMATION
Calories: 138, Fat: 2g, Saturated Fat: 0g, Cholesterol: 0mg, Fiber: 1g, Protein: 6g, Carbohydrate: 34g, Sugar: 15g, Sodium: 51mg

SUPER NUTRIENTS
Vitamin C: 173%, Vitamin K: 726%, Copper: 217%

Cleansing Lemonade

Lemons are detoxifying superstars. Enjoy this juice for a cleansing, immune-boosting kick.

INGREDIENTS

3 lemons
1 cucumber
1 apple, cored
½-inch piece ginger

Juice.

NUTRITIONAL INFORMATION
Calories: 102, Fat: 1g, Saturated Fat: 0g, Cholesterol: 0mg,
Fiber: 1g, Protein: 3g, Carbohydrate: 35g, Sugar: 18g, Sodium: 9mg

SUPER NUTRIENT
Vitamin C: 84%

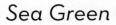

Sea Green

This powerful drink is packed full of iron and vitamin K, both of which are essential for healthy blood. Add a dash of kelp powder for an added mineral boost!

INGREDIENTS

8–10 carrots
1 small orange
1 bunch spinach
1 lemon
1 teaspoon kelp powder

Juice carrots, orange, spinach, and lemon. Stir in kelp powder.

NUTRITIONAL INFORMATION
Calories: 168, Fat: 0g, Saturated Fat: 0g, Cholesterol: 0mg, Fiber: 2g, Protein: 11g, Carbohydrate: 49g, Sugar: 23g, Sodium: 424mg

SUPER NUTRIENTS
Vitamin A: 441%, Vitamin C: 140%, Vitamin K: 990%, Folate: 136%, Iron: 96%

Note: Kelp powder is not included in analysis

Ravishing Radish

Radishes are natural liver cleansers! They increase bile flow and help to digest dietary fats. Enjoy this tasty juice anytime you need a little kick in your step!

INGREDIENTS

6 radishes, including leaves
1 small fennel bulb
6 celery stalks
1 cucumber
1 handful parsley
1 orange

Juice.

NUTRITIONAL INFORMATION
Calories: 107, *Fat:* 1g, *Saturated Fat:* 0g, *Cholesterol:* 0mg, *Fiber:* 2g, *Protein:* 6g, *Carbohydrate:* 25g, *Sugar:* 12g, *Sodium:* 165mg

SUPER NUTRIENTS
Vitamin B$_6$: 25%, *Vitamin C:* 123%, *Vitamin K:* 409%

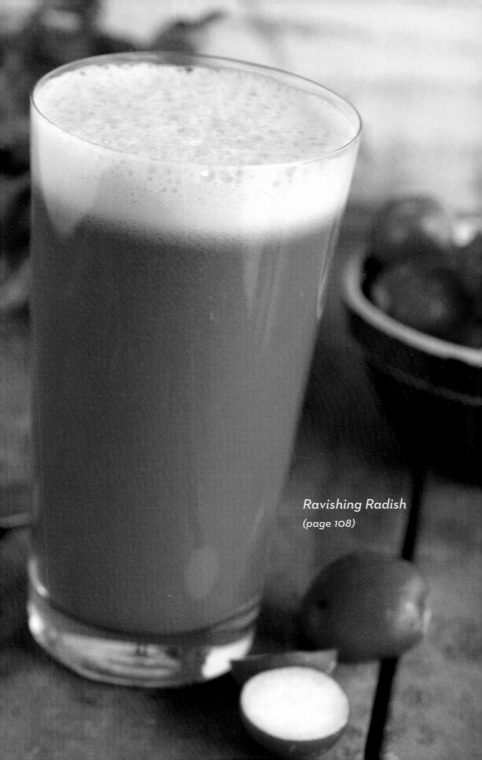

Ravishing Radish
(page 108)

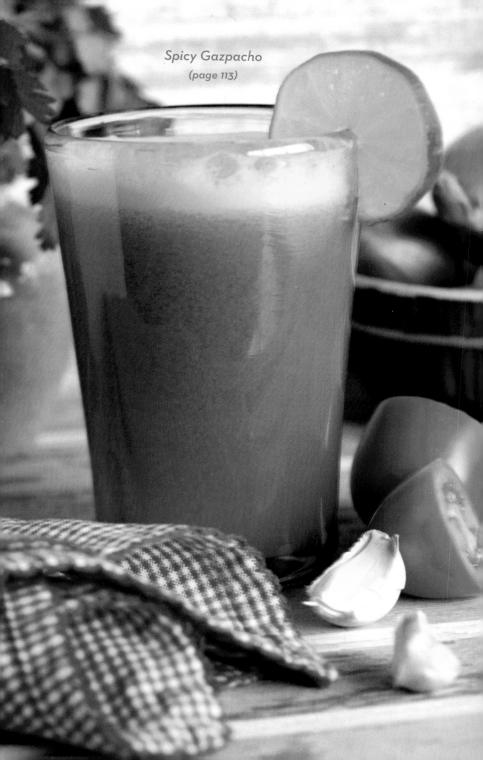

Spicy Gazpacho
(page 113)

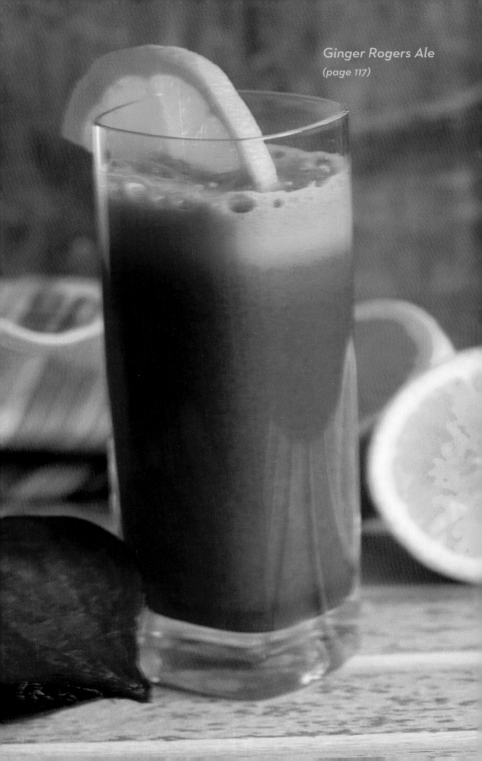

Ginger Rogers Ale
(page 117)

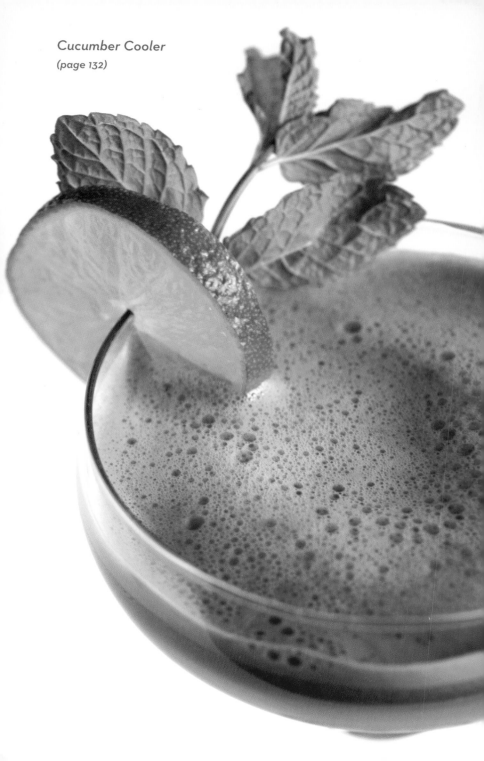

Cucumber Cooler
(page 132)

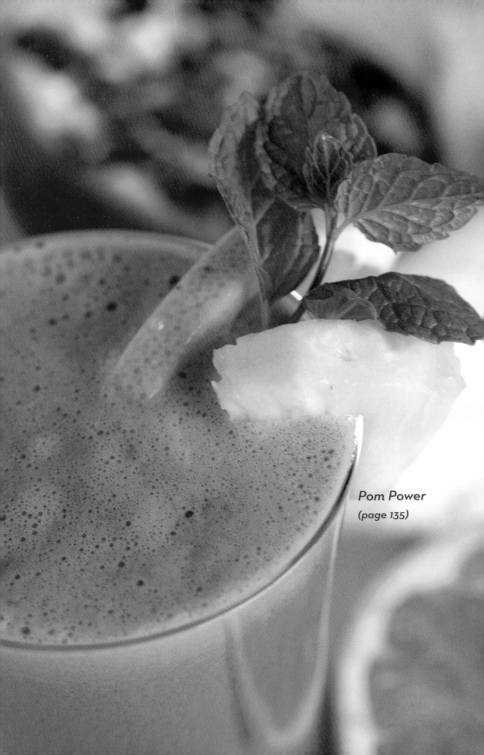

Pom Power
(page 135)

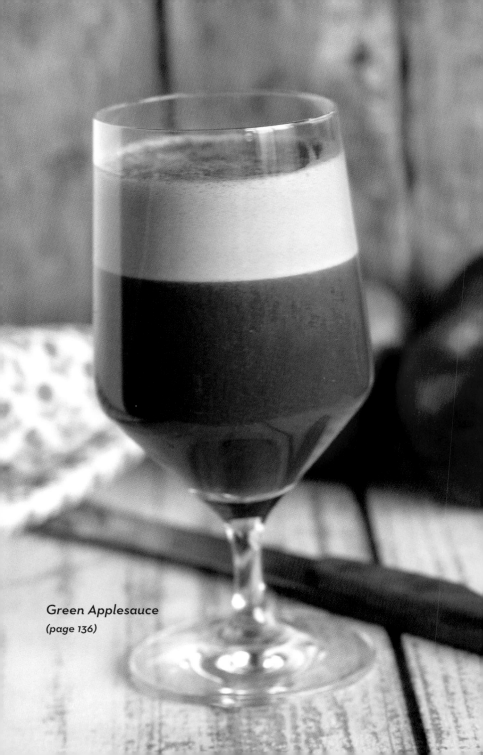

Green Applesauce
(page 136)

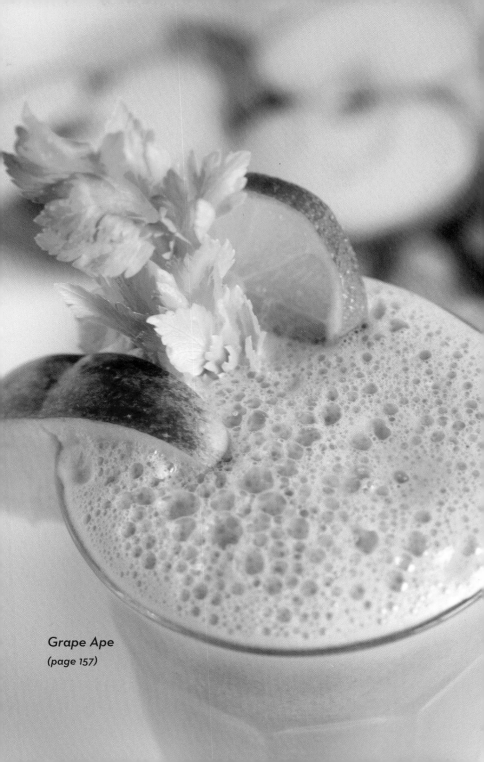

Grape Ape

(page 157)

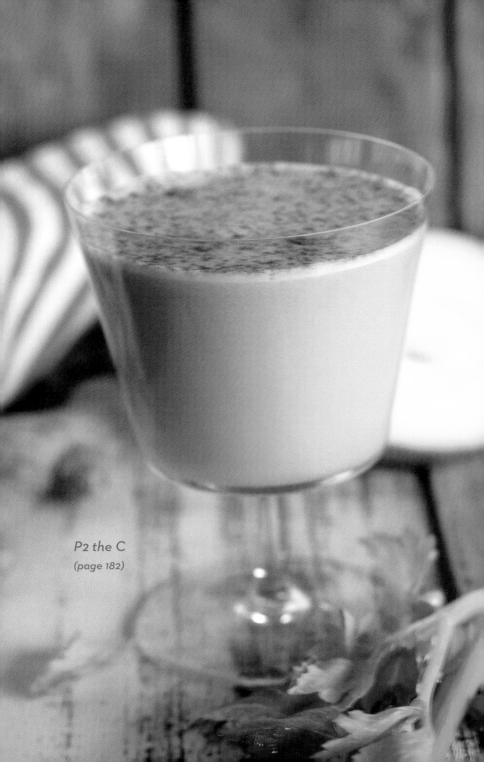

P2 the C
(page 182)

D-Tox Delight

Cleanse your body with every sip of this delicious juice. Loaded with vitamin A, an energizing beet, and hydrating cucumber, this juice is the perfect detox drink.

INGREDIENTS
4 carrots
2 celery stalks
1 cucumber
½ lemon
1 small beet
1 apple, cored

Juice.

NUTRITIONAL INFORMATION
Calories: 141, *Fat:* 1g, *Saturated Fat:* 0g, *Cholesterol:* 0mg, *Fiber:* 1g, *Protein:* 4g, *Carbohydrate:* 44g, *Sugar:* 26g, *Sodium:* 166mg

SUPER NUTRIENT
Vitamin A: 132%

Fly By Fennel

The combination of fennel, grapefruit, and mint is so liver supportive. Grapefruit is rich in antioxidants, fennel is a natural diuretic, and mint is one of the more effective herbs at promoting liver health.

INGREDIENTS
1 fennel bulb
½ grapefruit
1 cucumber
5–6 mint leaves
2 kale leaves

Juice.

NUTRITIONAL INFORMATION
Calories: 94, Fat: 0g, Saturated Fat: 0g, Cholesterol: 0mg, Fiber: 1g, Protein: 6g, Carbohydrate: 27g, Sugar: 6g, Sodium: 108mg

SUPER NUTRIENTS
Vitamin C: 107%, Vitamin K: 317%, Copper: 105%

Spicy Gazpacho

Cilantro is a natural cleansing agent. It promotes heavy metal detoxification by binding to and releasing heavy metals from cells. It also has amazing antioxidant and antimicrobial properties.

INGREDIENTS
2 tomatoes
2 cucumbers
1 bell pepper
1 shallot
1 garlic clove
1 handful fresh cilantro
1 lime

Juice.

NUTRITIONAL INFORMATION
Calories: 104, Fat: 1g, Saturated Fat: 0g, Cholesterol: 0mg, Fiber: 1g, Protein: 6g, Carbohydrate: 32g, Sugar: 14g, Sodium: 30mg

SUPER NUTRIENTS
Vitamin C: 103%, Vitamin K: 131%

Minty Mojito

Kale is the king of detox support. It contains compounds called glucosinolates that support liver detoxification at the cellular level. Drink this juice and give your body a leg up in eliminating toxic buildup.

INGREDIENTS
1 cucumber
1 handful mint, plus more for garnish
5 kale leaves
1 lime

Juice. Garnish with mint leaves.

NUTRITIONAL INFORMATION
Calories: 97, Fat: 1g, Saturated Fat: 0g, Cholesterol: 0mg, Fiber: 0g, Protein: 7g, Carbohydrate: 23g, Sugar: 4g, Sodium: 52mg

SUPER NUTRIENTS
Vitamin C: 185%, Vitamin K: 749%, Copper: 217%

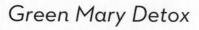

Green Mary Detox

Enjoy this healthy, detoxifying, low-sodium green drink anytime you're in the mood for something savory. Serve it with a celery stalk, dash of Tabasco sauce, and freshly ground pepper for a Green Mary mocktail!

INGREDIENTS

1 head romaine lettuce
2 tomatoes
2 celery stalks
1 scallion
2 carrots
1 lime

Juice.

NUTRITIONAL INFORMATION
Calories: 93, *Fat:* 2g, *Saturated Fat:* 0g, *Cholesterol:* 0mg, *Fiber:* 2g, *Protein:* 8g, Carbohydrate: 32g, *Sugar:* 13g, *Sodium:* 110mg

SUPER NUTRIENTS
Vitamin A: 284%, *Vitamin C:* 60%, *Vitamin K:* 402%, *Folate:* 161%, *Iron:* 65%

Dande-Mint

The apple, kiwi, and mint in this tangy juice do a great job toning down the bitterness of the liver-purifying dandelion greens. Dandelion is also a natural diuretic and helps to remove excess water and toxins from the body.

INGREDIENTS
1 large handful dandelion greens
½ cucumber
1 green apple, cored
1 kiwi, peeled
5–6 mint leaves

Juice.

NUTRITIONAL INFORMATION
Calories: 96, *Fat:* 1g, *Saturated Fat:* 0g, *Cholesterol:* 0mg, *Fiber:* 1g, *Protein:* 3g, *Carbohydrate:* 29g, *Sugar:* 17g, *Sodium:* 34mg

SUPER NUTRIENTS
Vitamin C: 73%, *Vitamin K:* 282%

Ginger Rogers Ale

This healthy and delicious take on ginger ale will help heal the digestive tract and support liver function, as it warms your body from the inside out.

INGREDIENTS
4 parsnips
1 beet
1 red bell pepper
1-inch piece ginger
1 orange

Juice.

NUTRITIONAL INFORMATION
Calories: 151, *Fat:* 1g, *Saturated Fat:* 0g, *Cholesterol:* 0mg, *Fiber:* 2g, *Protein:* 5g, *Carbohydrate:* 44g, *Sugar:* 22g, *Sodium:* 110mg

SUPER NUTRIENTS
Vitamin A: 188%, *Vitamin C:* 183%

Fennel of Love

Fennel helps promote digestion and is a natural diuretic. It's also an excellent source of potassium, which can help lower blood pressure.

INGREDIENTS
1 large fennel bulb
½ cucumber
½ green apple, cored
1 handful mint
1-inch piece ginger

Juice.

NUTRITIONAL INFORMATION
Calories: 81, *Fat:* 1g, *Saturated Fat:* 0g, *Cholesterol:* 0mg, *Fiber:* 1g, *Protein:* 3g, Carbohydrate: 26g, *Sugar:* 7g, *Sodium:* 90mg

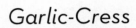

Garlic-Cress

Garlic is a detox superstar! It stimulates the liver to produce detoxification enzymes that help flush out toxins. It also contains allicin and selenium, two powerful nutrients shown to help protect the liver from toxic damage.

INGREDIENTS

2 carrots
1 cup chopped pineapple
1 small garlic clove
1 handful watercress
1-inch piece ginger
1 lemon

Juice.

NUTRITIONAL INFORMATION
Calories: 99, *Fat:* 1g, *Saturated Fat:* 0g, *Cholesterol:* 0mg, *Fiber:* 1g,
Protein: 3g, *Carbohydrate:* 30g, *Sugar:* 16g, *Sodium:* 63mg

SUPER NUTRIENTS
Vitamin A: 70%, *Vitamin C:* 103%

7

Juices for Weight Loss

Moji-cama

This mojito-inspired juice is my favorite treat on a warm summer day. Jicama and cucumber are both high in water and low in calories and sugar, making this juice a perfect complement to eating light.

INGREDIENTS
1 jicama, sliced
1 cucumber
3–5 collard leaves
1 handful mint
½ lime

Juice.

NUTRITIONAL INFORMATION
Calories: 90, *Fat:* 1g, *Saturated Fat:* 0g, *Cholesterol:* 0mg,
Fiber: 3g, *Protein:* 5g, *Carbohydrate:* 35g, *Sugar:* 8g, *Sodium:* 29mg

SUPER NUTRIENTS
Vitamin C: 82%, *Vitamin K:* 122%

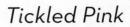

Tickled Pink

Get a blast of immune-boosting vitamin C and beta-carotene in this tasty pink drink.

INGREDIENTS

1 pink grapefruit
4 carrots
1-inch piece ginger
½ lemon

Juice.

NUTRITIONAL INFORMATION

Calories: 79, Fat: 1g, Saturated Fat: 0g, Cholesterol: 0mg, Fiber: 1g, Protein: 2g, Carbohydrate: 24g, Sugar: 12g, Sodium: 99mg

SUPER NUTRIENT

Vitamin A: 133%

O$_2$ Builder

Beets are the star in this ruby-red juice rich in antioxidants and naturally occurring nitrates. Nitrates help improve blood flow throughout the body and increase nitric oxide, which increases oxygen flow to your cells and lowers blood pressure. Try this delicious tonic before your morning workout for a boost of oxygen.

INGREDIENTS

2 beets
1 carrot
1 cup strawberries
1 apple, cored

Juice.

NUTRITIONAL INFORMATION
Calories: 99, *Fat:* 1g, *Saturated Fat:* 0g, *Cholesterol:* 0mg, *Fiber:* 1g, *Protein:* 3g, *Carbohydrate:* 32g, *Sugar:* 16g, *Sodium:* 139mg

Kiwi Kooler

This low-sugar drink is juice full of vitamin C, beta-carotene, and other immune-boosting compounds. Get your juice on for very little calories with this tasty treat!

INGREDIENTS
1 kiwi
1 cucumber
1 cup strawberries
½ lime
1 handful mint, plus more for garnish

Juice. Garnish with mint leaves.

NUTRITIONAL INFORMATION
Calories: 86, *Fat:* 2g, *Saturated Fat:* 0g, *Cholesterol:* 0mg,
Fiber: 1g, *Protein:* 3g, *Carbohydrate:* 27g, *Sugar:* 14g,
Sodium: 106mg

SUPER NUTRIENT
Vitamin C: 137%

Red Fresca

This is a natural energy drink! It has tons of antioxidant and anti-aging properties and the chia seeds pack an additional nutritious punch. They are a great source of fiber, protein, and essential omega-3 fats that will help keep you full!

INGREDIENTS
1 lemon
1 red apple, cored
1 red bell pepper
2–3 tablespoons chia seeds

Juice lemon, apple, and bell pepper. Stir in chia seeds. Let sit for a few minutes to thicken. Stir before drinking.

NUTRITIONAL INFORMATION
Calories: 133, *Fat:* 6g, *Saturated Fat:* 1g, *Cholesterol:* 0mg, *Fiber:* 2g, *Protein:* 4g, *Carbohydrate:* 30g, *Sugar:* 15g, *Sodium:* 6mg

SUPER NUTRIENT
Vitamin C: 147%

Green Machine

This low-calorie green juice is simple, yet satisfying. Great for a midmorning pick-me-up!

INGREDIENTS
3 Swiss chard leaves
3 celery stalks
1 cucumber
1 apple, cored
1 lime

Juice.

NUTRITIONAL INFORMATION
*Calories: 99, Fat: 1g, Saturated Fat: 0g, Cholesterol: 0mg, Fiber: 1g,
Protein: 4g, Carbohydrate: 32g, Sugar: 17g, Sodium: 249mg*

SUPER NUTRIENT
Vitamin K: 737%

Baby, I'm Amazed

This spicy green juice—with a little help from cayenne pepper—will get your metabolism humming!

INGREDIENTS
1 handful watercress
2 celery stalks
1 kiwi
½ grapefruit
1-inch piece ginger
1 lemon
Dash cayenne pepper

Juice.

NUTRITIONAL INFORMATION
Calories: 58, *Fat:* 1g, *Saturated Fat:* 0g, *Cholesterol:* 0mg, *Fiber:* 1g,
Protein: 2g, *Carbohydrate:* 18g, *Sugar:* 9g, *Sodium:* 28mg

Mint Extravaganza

This minty, low-calorie juice has just the right amount of sweet to satisfy any sugar cravings!

INGREDIENTS
1 large handful mint
2 cups chopped watermelon (peeled and seeded)
5–6 kale leaves
1 handful parsley

Juice.

NUTRITIONAL INFORMATION
Calories: 128, Fat: 2g, Saturated Fat: 0g, Cholesterol: 0mg,
Fiber: 2g, Protein: 7g, Carbohydrate: 29g, Sugar: 13g, Sodium: 64mg

SUPER NUTRIENTS
Vitamin C: 224%, Vitamin K: 1102%, Copper: 219%, Iron: 51%

Natural Born Pain Killer

This turmeric-spiked juice is a natural pain killer! Loaded with antioxidants and anti-inflammatory properties, it will ease the pain of that intense workout and provide a natural energy boost, too!

INGREDIENTS
3 celery stalks
1 cucumber
1 cup chopped pineapple
1 handful spinach
1-inch piece ginger
1-inch piece turmeric root, or a pinch turmeric powder

Juice. If using powdered turmeric, stir in.

NUTRITIONAL INFORMATION
Calories: 106, *Fat:* 1g, *Saturated Fat:* 0g, *Cholesterol:* 0mg, *Fiber:* 2g, *Protein:* 3g, *Carbohydrate:* 59g, *Sugar:* 18g, *Sodium:* 172mg

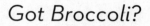

Got Broccoli?

Broccoli is the new milk. Loaded with vitamin C and just as much calcium per ounce as milk, this juice is good for your bones and your waistline.

INGREDIENTS
1 large head broccoli
1 cucumber
1 head romaine lettuce
1 red bell pepper
½ lemon

Juice.

NUTRITIONAL INFORMATION
Calories: 95, *Fat:* 2g, *Saturated Fat:* 0g, *Cholesterol:* 0mg, *Fiber:* 2g, *Protein:* 9g, *Carbohydrate:* 30g, *Sugar:* 12g, *Sodium:* 54mg

SUPER NUTRIENTS
Vitamin A: 224%, *Vitamin C:* 150%, *Vitamin K:* 438%, *Calcium:* 40%, *Folate:* 165%, *Iron:* 68%

Cucumber Cooler

The popular duo of watermelon and cucumber is perfect for rehydrating on a hot summer day. High in water and electrolytes, this juice balances the fluid levels in your body and keeps you cool . . . as a cucumber.

INGREDIENTS
2 cups chopped watermelon (peeled and seeded)
1 large cucumber
1 handful mint leaves
1–2 limes

Juice.

NUTRITIONAL INFORMATION
Calories: 98, *Fat:* 1g, *Saturated Fat:* 0g, *Cholesterol:* 0mg, *Fiber:* 1g, *Protein:* 3g, *Carbohydrate:* 29g, *Sugar:* 18g, *Sodium:* 7mg

You Say Tomato

This savory juice is a great midday snack. Chock-full of antioxidants and anti-cancer compounds, it's also a nutrition powerhouse. I like to serve it with chopped avocado.

INGREDIENTS
2–3 Roma tomatoes
2 zucchini
4 carrots
5–6 asparagus stalks
1 garlic clove

Juice.

NUTRITIONAL INFORMATION
Calories: 91, *Fat:* 1g, *Saturated Fat:* 0g, *Cholesterol:* 0mg, *Fiber:* 1g, *Protein:* 5g, *Carbohydrate:* 26g, *Sugar:* 15g, *Sodium:* 117mg

SUPER NUTRIENT
Vitamin A: 139%

Energize Tea

This simple juice-tea is great for a quick afternoon energy boost! Matcha is cleansing and adds extra antioxidants, fiber, and chlorophyll.

INGREDIENTS
1 apple, cored
1 fennel bulb
½ lemon
1 teaspoon matcha green tea powder

Juice apple, fennel, and lemon. Stir in matcha.

NUTRITIONAL INFORMATION
Calories: 92, *Fat:* 1g, *Saturated Fat:* 0g, *Cholesterol:* 0mg, *Fiber:* 1g, *Protein:* 2g, *Carbohydrate:* 21g, *Sugar:* 13g, *Sodium:* 87mg

Pom Power

This combination of romaine lettuce and fruit is refreshing and light. The pomegranate seeds provide antioxidant power and zing!

INGREDIENTS
½ head romaine lettuce
1 pink grapefruit
5–6 mint leaves
¼ cup pomegranate arils

Juice lettuce, grapefruit, and mint. Sprinkle pom arils on top for garnish.

NUTRITIONAL INFORMATION
Calories: 73, Fat: 1g, Saturated Fat: 0g, Cholesterol: 0mg, Fiber: 1g, Protein: 4g, Carbohydrate: 22g, Sugar: 15g, Sodium: 20mg

SUPER NUTRIENTS
Vitamin A: 116%, Vitamin K: 187%, Folate: 80%

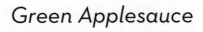

Green Applesauce

This is one of my favorite juice drinks for when I need a boost of energy in the afternoon. It tastes just like applesauce in a glass, and I love the added texture from the chia seeds!

INGREDIENTS
1 apple, cored
1 big handful spinach leaves
1 tablespoon chia seeds
Dash cinnamon

Juice apple and spinach and pour into glass. Stir in chia seeds and let sit for a few minutes to thicken. Serve with sprinkle of cinnamon.

NUTRITIONAL INFORMATION
Calories: 120, *Fat:* 5g, *Saturated Fat:* 0g, *Cholesterol:* 0mg, *Fiber:* 1g, *Protein:* 4g, *Carbohydrate:* 25g, *Sugar:* 13g, *Sodium:* 17mg

Jicama Fiesta

This gazpacho-inspired juice is light, refreshing, and delicious! Jicama is a sweet root vegetable with a clean, sweet flavor that makes a wonderful base for this savory juice. Garnish with chopped avocado for a balanced snack.

INGREDIENTS
1 small jicama
1 lime
2 tomatoes
1 garlic clove
½ avocado, chopped

Juice jicama, lime, tomatoes, and garlic. Garnish with some avocado.

NUTRITIONAL INFORMATION
Calories: 183, Fat: 10g, Saturated Fat: 2g, Cholesterol: 0mg, Fiber: 3g, Protein: 5g, Carbohydrate: 40g, Sugar: 10g, Sodium: 28mg

SUPER NUTRIENT
Vitamin C: 108%

Naturalizer

This refreshing dose of delicious natural energy will get you through that afternoon slump. Pear and strawberry combine with spinach to provide antioxidant-rich energy you need to feel revitalized!

INGREDIENTS

1 pear, cored
1 cup strawberries
1 handful spinach
Pinch cayenne pepper

Juice pear, strawberries, and spinach. Sprinkle with cayenne pepper.

NUTRITIONAL INFORMATION

Calories: 90, *Fat:* 1g, *Saturated Fat:* 0g, *Cholesterol:* 0mg, *Fiber:* 1g, *Protein:* 2g, *Carbohydrate:* 28g, *Sugar:* 17g, *Sodium:* 17mg

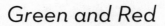

Green and Red

I love a simple, two-ingredient powerhouse juice. This combination will leave you feeling super-hydrated and vitalized!

INGREDIENTS
2–3 cups chopped watermelon (peeled and seeded)
1 large cucumber

Juice. Garnish glass with cucumber slices.

NUTRITIONAL INFORMATION
Calories: 89, *Fat:* 1g, *Saturated Fat:* 0g, *Cholesterol:* 0mg, *Fiber:* 0g, *Protein:* 3g, *Carbohydrate:* 24g, *Sugar:* 17g, *Sodium:* 6mg

Summer Sun

This unique juice is a perfect hydrator in the summertime—when tomatoes and watermelon are both in season. High in lycopene from the tomatoes, this juice contains natural cancer-fighting antioxidants plus a healthy dose of vitamin C and potassium.

INGREDIENTS
2 cups chopped watermelon (peeled and seeded)
2 Roma tomatoes
1 lime

Juice.

NUTRITIONAL INFORMATION
Calories: 88, *Fat:* 1g, *Saturated Fat:* 0g, *Cholesterol:* 0mg, *Fiber:* 1g, *Protein:* 3g, *Carbohydrate:* 26g, *Sugar:* 17g, *Sodium:* 9mg

Green Recovery

This green juice gets a tropical flair from coconut water and is the perfect electrolyte replacer after a sweaty workout.

INGREDIENTS
5 celery stalks
1 handful spinach
1 handful mint
1 lime
1–2 ounces unsweetened coconut water

Juice celery, spinach, mint, and lime. Stir in coconut water.

NUTRITIONAL INFORMATION
Calories: 40, *Fat:* 1g, *Saturated Fat:* 0g, *Cholesterol:* 0mg, *Fiber:* 1g, *Protein:* 2g, *Carbohydrate:* 13g, *Sugar:* 6g, *Sodium:* 214mg

Fuzzy Navel

This sweet juice is a delight! Simple yet nutrient-rich, it's a great low-calorie energy boost that will leave you feeling refreshed and invigorated.

INGREDIENTS
1 peach
1 handful spinach
2 zucchini

Juice.

NUTRITIONAL INFORMATION
Calories: 75, *Fat:* 1g, *Saturated Fat:* 0g, *Cholesterol:* 0mg, *Fiber:* 1g, *Protein:* 5g, *Carbohydrate:* 19g, *Sugar:* 16g, *Sodium:* 36mg

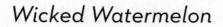

Wicked Watermelon

This light and hydrating drink will quench your thirst for something sweet and delicious!

INGREDIENTS
1 apple, cored
1 handful parsley
3 cups spinach
1 cup chopped watermelon (peeled and seeded)

Juice.

NUTRITIONAL INFORMATION
Calories: 92, Fat: 1g, Saturated Fat: 0g, Cholesterol: 0mg, Fiber: 1g, Protein: 4g, Carbohydrate: 27g, Sugar: 18g, Sodium: 68mg

SUPER NUTRIENT
Vitamin K: 638%

8

Super Immunity Juices

Flower Power

Cauliflower and broccoli are packed with vitamin C and tons of phytonutrients. This juice has a broad spectrum of anti-oxidant support that will keep your cells young, healthy, and alkalized.

INGREDIENTS
1 apple, cored
1 cup broccoli florets
4 carrots
2 cups chopped cauliflower
1-inch piece ginger

Juice.

NUTRITIONAL INFORMATION
Calories: 134, *Fat:* 1g, *Saturated Fat:* 0g, *Cholesterol:* 0mg, *Fiber:* 2g, *Protein:* 6g, *Carbohydrate:* 40g, *Sugar:* 21g, *Sodium:* 154mg

SUPER NUTRIENTS
Vitamin A: 131%, *Vitamin C:* 122%

Matcha Pear Tea

This energizing morning juice is loaded with concentrated antioxidants and vitamin C, which delivers a boost in absorption of green tea's powerful polyphenols. Upgrade your coffee and ward off disease with this tasty green tea.

INGREDIENTS

1 pear, cored
1 handful broccoli florets
3 carrots
1 cucumber
1 lemon, peeled
1 handful mint
1-inch piece ginger
Matcha green tea powder

Juice all ingredients except the matcha green tea powder. Stir in matcha.

NUTRITIONAL INFORMATION
Calories: 137, *Fat:* 1g, *Saturated Fat:* 0g, *Cholesterol:* 0mg, *Fiber:* 1g, *Protein:* 5g, *Carbohydrate:* 43g, *Sugar:* 21g, *Sodium:* 93mg

SUPER NUTRIENTS
Vitamin A: 100%, *Vitamin C:* 84%

Allergy Cure

Feeling the allergy blues? This powerhouse juice can ease those seasonal allergy symptoms with greens from the crucifer family as well as tons of vitamin C, beta-carotene, and other anti-inflammatory components.

INGREDIENTS

3 carrots
3 celery stalks
1 handful broccoli florets
5 kale leaves
3 collard leaves
1 garlic clove
2 oranges

Juice.

NUTRITIONAL INFORMATION
Calories: 165, Fat: 2g, Saturated Fat: 0g, Cholesterol: 0mg, Fiber: 1g, Protein: 10g, Carbohydrate: 42g, Sugar: 19g, Sodium: 165mg

SUPER NUTRIENTS
Vitamin A: 176%, Vitamin C: 300%, Vitamin K: 864%, Copper: 221%

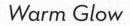

Warm Glow

This revved-up orange juice will warm you from the inside out on a cold winter morning. Highlighting only the orange, this juice is simple, healthy, and full of vitamin C. Garnish with a dash of cinnamon for an extra warming effect.

INGREDIENTS
2 oranges
1 lime
1-inch piece ginger
Dash cinnamon

Juice oranges, lime, and ginger. Top with a dash of cinnamon.

NUTRITIONAL INFORMATION
Calories: 74, *Fat:* 0g, *Saturated Fat:* 0g, *Cholesterol:* 0mg,
Fiber: 1g, *Protein:* 2g, *Carbohydrate:* 25g, *Sugar:* 14g, *Sodium:* 3mg

SUPER NUTRIENT
Vitamin C: 96%

Flu Schmoo

Give yourself a cellular tune-up with the immune-boosting, flu-fighting power of vitamins C and E and Spirulina.

INGREDIENTS
2 oranges
½ grapefruit
4 kale leaves
1-inch piece ginger
1 teaspoon Spirulina

Juice oranges, grapefruit, kale, and ginger. Stir in Spirulina.

NUTRITIONAL INFORMATION
Calories: 126, Fat: 1g, Saturated Fat: 0g, Cholesterol: 0mg, Fiber: 1g, Protein: 7g, Carbohydrate: 31g, Sugar: 15g, Sodium: 56mg

SUPER NUTRIENTS
Vitamin C: 225%, Vitamin K: 576%, Copper: 187%

Sweet Fennel

Fennel and orange come together well in this tasty juice that will help boost your immune system with tons of vitamin C.

INGREDIENTS
3 carrots
1 orange
1 small fennel bulb
½ lemon

Juice.

NUTRITIONAL INFORMATION
Calories: 95, Fat: 1g, Saturated Fat: 0g, Cholesterol: 0mg, Fiber: 2g, Protein: 4g, Carbohydrate: 32g, Sugar: 12g, Sodium: 158mg

SUPER NUTRIENT
Vitamin C: 130%

Peachy Keen

This juice is one of my favorite flavor combinations when I want the taste of fall in the summertime. The warming ginger and spicy cinnamon pair perfectly with the sweet taste of ripe peaches.

INGREDIENTS
2 sweet potatoes
1 peach
1-inch piece ginger
Sprinkle cinnamon

Juice potatoes, peach, and ginger. Top with a sprinkle of cinnamon.

NUTRITIONAL INFORMATION
Calories: 152, *Fat:* 1g, *Saturated Fat:* 0g, *Cholesterol:* 0mg, *Fiber:* 1g, *Protein:* 5g, *Carbohydrate:* 48g, *Sugar:* 11g, *Sodium:* 102mg

SUPER NUTRIENT
Vitamin A: 137%

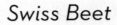

Swiss Beet

Step to the beet with this powerful drink! Beets and greens are heart-healthy duos that have been shown to help lower cholesterol and increase blood flow.

INGREDIENTS
2 beets
Handful parsley
5 Swiss chard leaves
1 cucumber
1 apple, cored

Juice.

NUTRITIONAL INFORMATION
Calories: 125, *Fat:* 1g, *Saturated Fat:* 0g, *Cholesterol:* 0mg, *Fiber:* 1g, *Protein:* 5g, *Carbohydrate:* 37g, *Sugar:* 23g, *Sodium:* 188mg

SUPER NUTRIENTS
Vitamin K: 645%, *Iron:* 50%

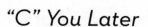

"C" You Later

This juice is loaded with the antioxidant and replenishing power of vitamin C. Enjoy this drink when you feel the sniffles coming on and jumpstart your immune system!

INGREDIENTS
2 Roma tomatoes
1 orange
1 cup strawberries
1 red bell pepper
2 carrots

Juice.

NUTRITIONAL INFORMATION
Calories: 102, *Fat:* 1g, *Saturated Fat:* 0g, *Cholesterol:* 0mg, *Fiber:* 1g, *Protein:* 4g, *Carbohydrate:* 30g, *Sugar:* 20g, *Sodium:* 58mg

SUPER NUTRIENT
Vitamin C: 203%

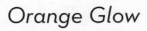

Orange Glow

Carrots and bell peppers are packed with beta-carotene, and turmeric adds an anti-inflammatory punch! This juice will help fight against free radicals and bring a healthy glow back to your skin.

INGREDIENTS
1 orange bell pepper
1 orange
1 carrot
1 small cucumber
1 lemon
Sprinkle turmeric powder

Juice bell pepper, orange, carrot, cucumber, and lemon. Sprinkle with turmeric.

NUTRITIONAL INFORMATION
Calories: 150, *Fat:* 1g, *Saturated Fat:* 0g, *Cholesterol:* 0mg, *Fiber:* 1g, *Protein:* 4g, *Carbohydrate:* 46g, *Sugar:* 23g, *Sodium:* 38mg

SUPER NUTRIENT
Vitamin C: 343%

Note: Turmeric powder not included in analysis

Citrus Delight

Both kiwi and oranges are excellent sources of vitamin C, which is a potent antioxidant. This juice is the perfect blend to give you nutrient-rich energy all morning.

INGREDIENTS
1 orange
1 kiwi
2 handfuls arugula
½ cucumber
1 lime
1 lemon

Juice.

NUTRITIONAL INFORMATION
Calories: 188, *Fat:* 1g, *Saturated Fat:* 0g, *Cholesterol:* 0mg, *Fiber:* 1g, *Protein:* 3g, *Carbohydrate:* 27g, *Sugar:* 15g, *Sodium:* 10mg

SUPER NUTRIENT
Vitamin C: 221%

Grape Ape

Grapes are wonderful full-body cleansers. They're packed with vitamins A, C, and folate. They also contain potassium and magnesium, which naturally reduce blood pressure, and resveratrol, a potent antioxidant and anti-ager.

INGREDIENTS
2 cups green grapes
2 celery sticks
½ cucumber
1 lime

Juice.

NUTRITIONAL INFORMATION
Calories: 98, Fat: 1g, Saturated Fat: 0g, Cholesterol: 0mg, Fiber: 1g, Protein: 3g, Carbohydrate: 28g, Sugar: 14g, Sodium: 24mg

Sweet and Spicy

Chard is one of the more detoxifying greens, mostly due to the compound betalain present in its red and yellow leaves. Betalain is great for detoxification as a potent antioxidant and anti-inflammatory.

INGREDIENTS
5–6 Swiss chard leaves
5–6 cilantro or parsley sprigs
1 carrot
1 green apple, cored
1 cucumber
1 lemon
1-inch piece ginger

Roll herbs into chard leaves. Juice all ingredients.

NUTRITIONAL INFORMATION
Calories: 159, *Fat:* 1g, *Saturated Fat:* 0g, *Cholesterol:* 0mg, *Fiber:* 2g, *Protein:* 7g, *Carbohydrate:* 49g, *Sugar:* 16g, *Sodium:* 163mg

SUPER NUTRIENTS
Vitamin C: 100%, *Vitamin K:* 1189%

'Flammation Fighter

Get armed and ready to fight inflammation and free radicals. Aloe juice fills this drink with all types of nutrients including vitamin B_{12}, essential amino acids, and antioxidants as well as hydration.

INGREDIENTS
2 cucumbers
3 celery stalks
1 apple, cored
5 kale leaves
1–2 ounces aloe vera juice

Juice cucumbers, celery, apple, and kale. Stir in aloe vera juice.

NUTRITIONAL INFORMATION
Calories: 165, *Fat:* 2g, *Saturated Fat:* 0g, *Cholesterol:* 0mg,
Fiber: 1g, *Protein:* 9g, *Carbohydrate:* 41g, *Sugar:* 16g, *Sodium:* 85mg

SUPER NUTRIENTS
Vitamin C: 183%, *Vitamin K:* 788%, *Copper:* 228%, *Iron:* 40%

Note: Aloe vera juice not included in analysis.

Taste of Thai

This spicy taste of Thailand is an antioxidant wonder. Broccoli sprouts, garlic, and kale offer up their concentrated protection in a tasty juice from the Far East.

INGREDIENTS
2 cucumbers
1 lime
1 handful basil
5 kale leaves
1 handful broccoli sprouts
1-inch piece ginger
1 garlic clove

Juice.

NUTRITIONAL INFORMATION
Calories: 142, *Fat:* 2g, *Saturated Fat:* 0g, *Cholesterol:* 0mg, *Fiber:* 1g, *Protein:* 9g, *Carbohydrate:* 35g, *Sugar:* 8g, *Sodium:* 59mg

SUPER NUTRIENTS
Vitamin C: 195%, *Vitamin K:* 808%, *Copper:* 235%

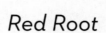

Red Root

This veggie delight will kick start your immune system and infuse your cells with the antioxidant power of beta-carotene.

INGREDIENTS
1 beet
1 carrot
1 sweet potato
1-inch piece ginger

Juice.

NUTRITIONAL INFORMATION
Calories: 175, *Fat:* 1g, *Saturated Fat:* 0g, *Cholesterol:* 0mg, *Fiber:* 2g, *Protein:* 4g, *Carbohydrate:* 40g, *Sugar:* 15g, *Sodium:* 160mg

SUPER NUTRIENT
Vitamin A: 234%

9

Juices for Anti-Aging and Glowing Skin

Radiance

The skin-loving power of cucumber and mango make this vitamin A–rich juice your skin's best friend. Replenish dull skin with this complexion elixir.

INGREDIENTS
½ cup mango, peeled and pitted
1 handful spinach
1 cucumber
1 tablespoon unsweetened shredded coconut

Juice mango, spinach, and cucumber. Stir in the shredded coconut.

NUTRITIONAL INFORMATION
Calories: 62, *Fat:* 0.5g, *Saturated Fat:* 4g, *Cholesterol:* 0mg, *Fiber:* 1g, *Protein:* 2g, *Carbohydrate:* 17g, *Sugar:* 15g, *Sodium:* 19mg

SUPER NUTRIENT
Vitamin K: 101%

Note: Shredded coconut not included in analysis.

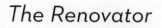

The Renovator

This tasty juice will renovate your skin with hydration and the antioxidant power of beta-carotene and vitamin C.

INGREDIENTS
1 fennel bulb
3 carrots
2 celery stalks
3–4 slices cantaloupe (peeled and seeded)
1 handful mint
1 lime

Juice.

NUTRITIONAL INFORMATION
Calories: 112, *Fat:* 1g, *Saturated Fat:* 0g, *Cholesterol:* 0mg, *Fiber:* 2g, *Protein:* 4g, *Carbohydrate:* 37g, *Sugar:* 15g, *Sodium:* 196mg

SUPER NUTRIENTS
Vitamin A: 120%, *Vitamin C:* 92%, *Iron:* 26%, *Potassium:* 31%

Purify

This simple vegetable tonic will keep your complexion glowing and your skin supple. Garnish with some pomegranate seeds for a sweet crunch, if desired.

INGREDIENTS
3 cucumbers
2 lemons
1 small head romaine lettuce
1 handful mint

Juice.

NUTRITIONAL INFORMATION
Calories: 140, *Fat:* 2g, *Saturated Fat:* 0g, Cholesterol: 0mg, *Fiber:* 2g, *Protein:* 10g, *Carbohydrate:* 45g, *Sugar:* 18g, *Sodium:* 49mg

SUPER NUTRIENTS
Vitamin A: 216%, *Vitamin C:* 87%, *Vitamin K:* 461%, *Folate:* 162%, *Iron:* 81%

Heart Strong

This mix of flavors is both heart healthy and bone smart. Bok choy is a great source of absorbable calcium and helps to lower cholesterol.

INGREDIENTS
2 carrots
1 apple, cored
4 kale leaves
1 handful basil
1 leek
1 baby bok choy
½ lemon, peeled

Juice.

NUTRITIONAL INFORMATION
Calories: 165, Fat: 2g, Saturated Fat: 0g, Cholesterol: 0mg, Fiber: 2g, Protein: 7g, Carbohydrate: 44g, Sugar: 16g, Sodium: 124mg

SUPER NUTRIENTS
Vitamin A: 223%, Vitamin C: 217%, Vitamin K: 644%, Copper: 184%

Berry Delicious

Simple and delicious, nutrient-rich juice will leave you feeling well fueled, yet light on your feet.

INGREDIENTS
1 apple, cored
2 cups strawberries
5 kale leaves
1 cucumber

Juice.

NUTRITIONAL INFORMATION
Calories: 183, *Fat:* 2g, *Saturated Fat:* 0g, *Cholesterol:* 0mg, *Fiber:* 3g, *Protein:* 8g, *Carbohydrate:* 48g, *Sugar:* 24g, *Sodium:* 54mg

SUPER NUTRIENTS
Vitamin C: 315%, *Vitamin K:* 754%, *Copper:* 228%

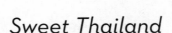

Sweet Thailand

In addition to being a light and refreshing treat on a hot summer day, this juice delivers a hefty shot of bone-protective vitamin K and potassium.

INGREDIENTS
1 cup chopped honeydew melon (peeled and seeded)
1 handful basil
1 cucumber
1 lime, peeled
1 handful cilantro
1-inch piece ginger

Juice.

NUTRITIONAL INFORMATION
Calories: 120, *Fat:* 1g, *Saturated Fat:* 0g, *Cholesterol:* 0mg, *Fiber:* 1g, *Protein:* 4g, *Carbohydrate:* 28g, *Sugar:* 16g, *Sodium:* 61mg

SUPER NUTRIENTS
Vitamin C: 79%, *Vitamin K:* 127%

Coco-loupe

Stuck in front of the computer all day? Give your eyes the support they need with this hydrating juice! Cantaloupe is rich in vitamin C and beta-carotene, essential nutrients that protect and preserve your overall eye health.

INGREDIENTS

1 cup chopped cantaloupe (peeled and seeded)
1 handful basil
1 head romaine lettuce
1 cucumber
1 tablespoon unsweetened shredded coconut

Juice cantaloupe, basil, romaine, and cucumber. Garnish with coconut flakes.

NUTRITIONAL INFORMATION
Calories: 110, Fat: 1g, Saturated Fat: 0g, Cholesterol: 0mg,
Fiber: 2g, Protein: 5g, Carbohydrate: 20g, Sugar: 16g, Sodium: 75mg

SUPER NUTRIENTS
Vitamin A: 217%, Vitamin C: 99%, Vitamin K: 438%, Folate: 166%,
Iron: 60%

Note: Coconut flakes not included in analysis.

Bone Up

Thanks to all the vitamin-rich greens, this juice is a bone-building powerhouse!

INGREDIENTS
1 handful broccoli florets
1 handful watercress
1 handful spinach
3 collard greens
1 cucumber
1-inch piece of ginger
2 oranges

Juice.

NUTRITIONAL INFORMATION
Calories: 109, *Fat:* 1g, *Saturated Fat:* 0g, *Cholesterol:* 0mg,
Fiber: 1g, *Protein:* 5g, *Carbohydrate:* 31g, *Sugar:* 17g, *Sodium:* 41mg

SUPER NUTRIENTS
Vitamin C: 145%, *Vitamin K:* 242%

Honey Boo-Boo

Honeydew is a great source of collagen-boosting vitamin C. This detoxifying and anti-aging juice is perfect on a warm summer day!

INGREDIENTS

1 cup chopped honeydew melon (peeled and seeded)
1 handful cilantro
1 lime

Juice.

NUTRITIONAL INFORMATION

Calories: 42, Fat: 0g, Saturated Fat: 0g, Cholesterol: 0mg, Fiber: 1g, Protein: 1g, Carbohydrate: 12g, Sugar: 10g, Sodium: 32mg

SUPER NUTRIENTS

Vitamin C: 58%, Vitamin K: 169%

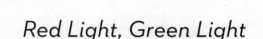

Red Light, Green Light

Simple and tasty, this juice is a great cleanser and revitalizer. Beet juice helps you glow from the inside out.

INGREDIENTS
2 beets
1 cucumber
1 red apple, cored
1-inch piece ginger
1 lime

Juice.

NUTRITIONAL INFORMATION
Calories: 105, Fat: 1g, Saturated Fat: 0g, Cholesterol: 0mg, Fiber: 1g, Protein: 3g, Carbohydrate: 30g, Sugar: 16g, Sodium: 52mg

Sassy Po-Tassy

This heart-healthy juice provides half a day's worth of potassium in one tasty glass!

INGREDIENTS
1 sweet potato
1 handful spinach
1-inch piece ginger
1 cup chopped cantaloupe (peeled and seeded)

Juice.

NUTRITIONAL INFORMATION
Calories: 153, Fat: 1g, Saturated Fat: 1g, Cholesterol: 0mg, Fiber: 2g, Protein: 9g, Carbohydrate: 39g, Sugar: 14g, Sodium: 259mg

SUPER NUTRIENTS
Vitamin A: 218%, Vitamin C: 123%, Folate: 124%, Iron: 91%

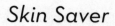

Skin Saver

The antioxidant power of carrots, orange, and cucumber is great for glowing skin!

INGREDIENTS
1 carrot
1 orange
1 cucumber
3 stalks celery

Juice.

NUTRITIONAL INFORMATION
Calories: 70, *Fat:* 1g, *Saturated Fat:* 0g, *Cholesterol:* 0mg,
Fiber: 0.5g, *Protein:* 3g, *Carbohydrate:* 20g, *Sugar:* 12g,
Sodium: 131mg

Green Sunscreen

Broccoli and carrots join forces in this sweet juice to provide the skin-protective power of vitamin A! Your skin will say thank you after sipping this anti-aging delight.

INGREDIENTS
1 handful spinach
3 broccoli stalks
3 large carrots
1 handful mint
1 apple, cored

Juice.

NUTRITIONAL INFORMATION
Calories: 97, *Fat:* 1g, *Saturated Fat:* 0g, *Cholesterol:* 0mg, *Fiber:* 3g, *Protein:* 4g, *Carbohydrate:* 30g, *Sugar:* 17g, *Sodium:* 293mg

SUPER NUTRIENTS
Vitamin C: 120%, *Vitamin K:* 166%

Age Defyer

Ignite your health with this spicy juice. Vitamins K and C combine to protect and restore your body at the cellular level.

INGREDIENTS

1 cucumber
1 pear
1 lemon
5 kale leaves
1-inch piece ginger

Juice.

NUTRITIONAL INFORMATION
Calories: 155, *Fat:* 2g, *Saturated Fat:* 0g, *Cholesterol:* 0mg,
Fiber: 1g, *Protein:* 8g, *Carbohydrate:* 41g, *Sugar:* 15g, *Sodium:* 55mg

SUPER NUTRIENTS
Vitamin C: 200%, *Vitamin K:* 752%, *Copper:* 229%

Skin Secret Sauce

Cucumbers are the fountain of youth for your skin. They are rich in hydrating nutrients and silica, which adds tone and elasticity to your complexion. Most of the silica is found in the peel, so it's best not to peel your cucumbers before juicing. Drink this skin tonic daily for smooth skin!

INGREDIENTS
1 apple, cored
2 celery stalks
3 cucumbers

Juice.

NUTRITIONAL INFORMATION
Calories: 131, *Fat:* 1g, *Saturated Fat:* 0g, *Cholesterol:* 0mg, *Fiber:* 1g, *Protein:* 5g, *Carbohydrate:* 38g, *Sugar:* 22g, *Sodium:* 33mg

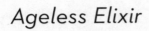

Ageless Elixir

Pineapple and cucumber work together to hydrate and nourish the skin. Pineapple juice also helps in the synthesis of collagen, which keeps skin smooth and supple. This simple juice will help keep you feeling and looking younger.

INGREDIENTS
1 cup chopped pineapple
1 handful parsley
1 cucumber

Juice.

NUTRITIONAL INFORMATION
Calories: 86, *Fat:* 1g, *Saturated Fat:* 0g, *Cholesterol:* 0mg, *Fiber:* 1g, *Protein:* 3g, *Carbohydrate:* 25g, *Sugar:* 15g, *Sodium:* 21mg

SUPER NUTRIENTS
Vitamin C: 109%, *Vitamin K:* 412%

Cabbage Crazy

Cabbage can help slow the aging process and keep skin healthy and young. It's rich in beta-carotene, vitamin C, and selenium, all three of which are powerful antioxidants and anti-inflammatory nutrients.

INGREDIENTS

4 large cabbage leaves

3 carrots

1 cucumber

1–inch piece of ginger

Juice.

NUTRITIONAL INFORMATION

Calories: 79, *Fat:* 1g, *Saturated Fat:* 0g, *Cholesterol:* 0mg, *Fiber:* 1g, *Protein:* 3g, *Carbohydrate:* 23g, *Sugar:* 10g, *Sodium:* 86mg

SUPER NUTRIENT

Vitamin A: 99%

10

Juices for
Digestive Health

P2 the C

This delicious juice is sweet, spicy, and soothing, thanks to the warming effect of the ginger and cinnamon. Super easy to digest, this comforting juice will keep your digestive tract humming!

INGREDIENTS
2 parsnips
1 pear, cored
2 celery stalks
1-inch piece ginger
Dash nutmeg or cinnamon

Juice parsnips, pear, celery, and ginger. Sprinkle with cinnamon or nutmeg.

NUTRITIONAL INFORMATION
Calories: 128, *Fat:* 1g, *Saturated Fat:* 0g, *Cholesterol:* 0mg, *Fiber:* 1g, *Protein:* 1g, *Carbohydrate:* 21g, *Sugar:* 17g, *Sodium:* 58mg

SUPER NUTRIENT
Calcium: 70%

Gut Soother

This sweet juice is great for soothing and healing the stomach, thanks to the fennel and ginger. Natural digestive aids, both can help reduce pain and decrease inflammation.

INGREDIENTS
1 fennel bulb
1 small apple, cored
1 small cucumber
1-inch piece ginger
1 head romaine lettuce

Juice.

NUTRITIONAL INFORMATION
Calories: 159, *Fat:* 2g, *Saturated Fat:* 0g, *Cholesterol:* 0mg,
Fiber: 3g, *Protein:* 9g, *Carbohydrate:* 51g, *Sugar:* 18g,
Sodium: 128mg

SUPER NUTRIENTS
Vitamin A: 214%, *Vitamin K:* 405%, *Folate:* 165%, *Iron:* 78%

Mornin' Glory

This restorative juice is the perfect breakfast drink for a boost of natural energy and healing power. Ginger and cayenne will wake up your digestive system and also help relieve gas and indigestion.

INGREDIENTS
1 cucumber
1 green apple, cored
1 lemon
5 kale leaves
1-inch piece ginger
Dash cayenne pepper

Juice cucumber, apple, lemon, kale, and ginger. Stir in cayenne pepper.

NUTRITIONAL INFORMATION
Calories: 153, Fat: 2g, Saturated Fat: 0g, Cholesterol: 0mg, Fiber: 1g, Protein: 8g, Carbohydrate: 40g, Sugar: 16g, Sodium: 55mg

SUPER NUTRIENTS
Vitamin C: 200%, Vitamin K: 750%, Copper: 223%

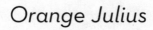

Orange Julius

Aloe vera helps to balance acid and alkaline levels in the stomach and ease gut irritation. It's also a potent antifungal, antiviral, and anti-inflammatory. It's a wonderful addition to this juice for creating optimal digestive and colon health.

INGREDIENTS

2 oranges, peeled
1 big handful spinach
1 ounce aloe vera juice

Juice oranges and spinach. Stir in aloe vera juice.

NUTRITIONAL INFORMATION

Calories: 54, Fat: 0g, Saturated Fat: 0g, Cholesterol: 0mg,
Fiber: 1g, Protein: 2g, Carbohydrate: 16g, Sugar: 13g, Sodium: 14mg

Note: Aloe vera juice not included in analysis.

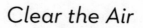

Clear the Air

This mix of mint, papaya, broccoli, and ginger is great for enhancing digestion. Papaya contains the enzyme papain, which helps digest proteins. High in vitamin C, it will also keep your gut healthy and strong.

INGREDIENTS

2 celery stalks
1 kale leaf
2–3 broccoli stems
½ papaya
½-inch piece ginger
½ lemon
1 handful mint

Juice.

NUTRITIONAL INFORMATION
Calories: 133, *Fat:* 2g, *Saturated Fat:* 0g, *Cholesterol:* 0mg, *Fiber:* 1g, *Protein:* 11g, *Carbohydrate:* 36g, *Sugar:* 11g, *Sodium:* 140mg

SUPER NUTRIENTS
Vitamin C: 409%, *Vitamin K:* 419 %, *Folate:* 60%

Red Reviver

This sweet and sassy juice will keep your digestive tract healthy. Both red grapes and red cabbage are potent antioxidants and have anti-aging, anticancer, anti-inflammation and antiviral properties.

INGREDIENTS
1 cup red grapes
¼ red cabbage
5 broccoli stems
3 celery stalks

Juice.

NUTRITIONAL INFORMATION
Calories: 195, *Fat:* 3g, *Saturated Fat:* 0g, *Cholesterol:* 0mg, *Fiber:* 3g, *Protein:* 16g, *Carbohydrate:* 55g, *Sugar:* 13g, *Sodium:* 1276mg

SUPER NUTRIENTS
Vitamin B$_6$: 95%, Vitamin C: 552%, Vitamin K: 507%, Folate: 76%, Iron: 64%

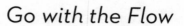

Go with the Flow

Pear is a natural digestive tract healer. It's a great source of pectin, which keeps things moving in the right direction. Stir in a bit of flax oil for an added boost of fiber!

INGREDIENTS
1 cucumber
2 celery stalks
1 pear, cored
1 kiwi
4 kale leaves
½ lemon
1–2 teaspoons flax oil

Juice all ingredients except the flax oil. Stir flax oil into juice.

NUTRITIONAL INFORMATION
Calories: 154, *Fat:* 2g, *Saturated Fat:* 0g, *Cholesterol:* 0mg, *Fiber:* 1g, *Protein:* 7g, *Carbohydrate:* 42g, *Sugar:* 19g, *Sodium:* 63mg

SUPER NUTRIENTS
Vitamin C: 205%, *Vitamin K:* 630%, *Copper:* 191%

Note: Flax oil not included in analysis.

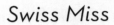

Swiss Miss

Swiss chard is working overtime in this juice, keeping your gut healthy *and* cancer free. Its high levels of anthocyanins have been shown to prevent cancers of the digestive tract.

INGREDIENTS
5 leaves rainbow Swiss chard
2 stalks celery
1 cucumber
1 cup chopped pineapple
1-inch piece ginger

Juice.

NUTRITIONAL INFORMATION
Calories: 117, *Fat:* 1g, *Saturated Fat:* 0g, *Cholesterol:* 0mg, *Fiber:* 1g,
Protein: 5g, *Carbohydrate:* 33g, *Sugar:* 17g, *Sodium:* 384mg

SUPER NUTRIENTS
Vitamin C: 126%, *Vitamin K:* 1197%, *Iron:* 51%

Smooth Sailin'

This sweet and creamy juice will go down smoothly. Sweet potatoes are great source of beta-carotene and the red pepper adds some vitamin C. The ginger keeps it warm and is great for digestion!

INGREDIENTS
1 sweet potato
1 carrot
1 red bell pepper
1-inch piece ginger

Juice.

NUTRITIONAL INFORMATION
Calories: 123, Fat: 1g, Saturated Fat: 0g, Cholesterol: 0mg, Fiber: 1g, Protein: 3g, Carbohydrate: 39g, Sugar: 13g, Sodium: 133mg

SUPER NUTRIENT
Vitamin A: 117%

Piña Colada

This tropical juice is a potent healer of the digestion system. Cabbage juice is the star, rich in sulforaphane, which helps to balance the bacteria in the gut and soothe stomach ulcers. Cabbage juice also contains the amino acid glutamine, which is healing and regenerating for the gut.

INGREDIENTS
1 orange
1 cup chopped pineapple
1 handful mint
½ jicama
½ savoy cabbage

Juice.

NUTRITIONAL INFORMATION
Calories: 104, *Fat:* 0g, *Saturated Fat:* 0g, *Cholesterol:* 0mg, *Fiber:* 1g, *Protein:* 2g, *Carbohydrate:* 34g, *Sugar:* 20g, *Sodium:* 6mg

SUPER NUTRIENT
Vitamin C: 130%

Dreamsicle

Travel back to your childhood with this dreamy juice. Orange, zucchini, and romaine pair up with a dash of vanilla extract to create this healthy alternative to the ice cream man!

INGREDIENTS
1 orange, peeled
2 zucchini
1 head romaine lettuce
Dash vanilla extract

Juice orange, zucchini, and romaine. Add vanilla extract.

NUTRITIONAL INFORMATION
Calories: 95, *Fat:* 1g, *Saturated Fat:* 0g, *Cholesterol:* 0mg, *Fiber:* 2g, *Protein:* 4g, *Carbohydrate:* 29g, *Sugar:* 16g, *Sodium:* 48mg

SUPER NUTRIENTS
Vitamin A: 216%, *Vitamin C:* 132%, *Vitamin K:* 380%, *Folate:* 169%, *Iron:* 62%

11

Cancer-Fighting Juices

Spicy Sprouts

The cancer-fighting duo of kale and broccoli sprouts make this spicy juice a mighty drink! Both contain powerful antioxidants that protect our cells from free radical damage and help ward off breast, colon, ovarian, prostate, and bladder cancer.

INGREDIENTS
1 handful broccoli sprouts
5 kale leaves
1 small apple, cored
1 handful cilantro
2 cucumbers
1-inch piece ginger

Fold sprouts into kale leaves and juice along with all the other ingredients.

NUTRITIONAL INFORMATION
Calories: 188, *Fat:* 3g, *Saturated Fat:* 1g, *Cholesterol:* 0mg, *Fiber:* 1g, *Protein:* 10g, *Carbohydrate:* 46g, *Sugar:* 18g, *Sodium:* 70mg

SUPER NUTRIENTS
Vitamin C: 222%, *Vitamin K:* 984%, *Copper:* 262%, *Iron:* 48%

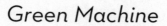

Green Machine

This team of green has got your back! Chock-full of anti-oxidants and cancer-fighting nutrients, a glass each day will keep the doctor away.

INGREDIENTS
3 collard green leaves
1 green apple, cored
1 cucumber
2–3 handfuls of spinach
1 handful cilantro
½ lime

Juice.

NUTRITIONAL INFORMATION
Calories: 99, Fat: 1g, Saturated Fat: 0g, Cholesterol: 0mg, Fiber: 1g, Protein: 6g, Carbohydrate: 31g, Sugar: 15g, Sodium: 57mg

SUPER NUTRIENT
Vitamin K: 509%

Greek Goodness

I love the taste of this Greek-inspired, cancer-fighting juice; it's like salad in a glass!

INGREDIENTS
3 Roma tomatoes
1 bell pepper
1 handful spinach
1 handful basil
1 garlic clove
½ head romaine lettuce

Juice.

NUTRITIONAL INFORMATION
Calories: 66, *Fat:* 1g, *Saturated Fat:* 0g, *Cholesterol:* 0mg, *Fiber:* 1g, *Protein:* 6g, *Carbohydrate:* 19g, *Sugar:* 10g, *Sodium:* 44mg

SUPER NUTRIENTS
Vitamin A: 136%, *Vitamin C:* 120%, *Vitamin K:* 303%, Folate 98%, *Iron:* 46%

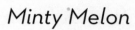

Minty Melon

Watermelon is perfect for juicing and for weight loss! Being more than 90 percent water, this melon has fewer calories per serving than most other fruits. It's also a great source of lycopene, a powerful antioxidant with anti-cancer properties.

INGREDIENTS
2 cups chopped watermelon (peeled and seeded)
½ cucumber
2–3 kale leaves
5–6 fresh mint leaves
1 lime

Juice.

NUTRITIONAL INFORMATION
Calories: 108, *Fat:* 1g, *Saturated Fat:* 0g, *Cholesterol:* 0mg, *Fiber:* 0g, *Protein:* 4g, *Carbohydrate:* 29g, *Sugar:* 16g, *Sodium:* 24mg

SUPER NUTRIENTS
Vitamin C: 103%, *Vitamin K:* 303%, *Copper:* 100%

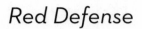

Red Defense

This juice is loaded with cancer-fighting lycopene, antioxidants, and soluble fiber. The reishi mushroom extract adds an extra shot of protection by revving up your immunity and calming inflammation.

INGREDIENTS

**1 apple, cored
1 cup strawberries
1 cucumber
1 small head broccoli
Few drops reishi mushroom extract**

Juice apple, strawberries, cucumber, and broccoli. Add a few drops reishi extract and stir.

NUTRITIONAL INFORMATION
Calories: 128, *Fat:* 1g, *Saturated Fat:* 0g, *Cholesterol:* 0mg,
Fiber: 2g, *Protein:* 4g, *Carbohydrate:* 41g, *Sugar:* 18g, *Sodium:* 15mg

SUPER NUTRIENT
Vitamin C: 126%

Note: Reishi extract not included in analysis.

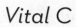

Vital C

This lycopene- and antioxidant-rich juice is a great cancer fighter, anti-ager, and immune booster. It's your daily shot of health!

INGREDIENTS
2 red bell peppers
3 Roma tomatoes
3 carrots
1 handful parsley or basil

Juice.

NUTRITIONAL INFORMATION
Calories: 90, *Fat:* 1g, *Saturated Fat:* 0g, *Cholesterol:* 0mg, *Fiber:* 1g, *Protein:* 5g, *Carbohydrate:* 26g, *Sugar:* 15g, *Sodium:* 102mg

SUPER NUTRIENTS
Vitamin A: 138%, *Vitamin C:* 224%, *Vitamin K:* 411%

Power House

Mango has recently been added to the list of cancer-fighting fruits. Pair it with the nutrition power of broccoli and spinach for a delicious anti-cancer infusion.

INGREDIENTS

1 mango
1 cucumber
2–3 broccoli stems
2 cups spinach

Juice.

NUTRITIONAL INFORMATION
Calories: 214, *Fat:* 2g, *Saturated Fat:* 0g, *Cholesterol:* 0mg, *Fiber:* 2g, *Protein:* 10g, *Carbohydrate:* 58g, *Sugar:* 39g, *Sodium:* 110mg

SUPER NUTRIENTS
Vitamin B_6: 63%, Vitamin C: 324%, Vitamin K: 385%, Folate: 83%, Iron: 46%

Blue Love

This blue juice is a potent antioxidant elixir. The pineapple provides vitamin C and potassium and the blueberries contain tons of anthocyanins, which are potent cancer fighters.

INGREDIENTS
½ cup pineapple
1 cucumber
5–6 kale leaves
1 cup blueberries
1-inch piece ginger

Juice.

NUTRITIONAL INFORMATION
Calories: 176, *Fat:* 1g, *Saturated Fat:* 0g, *Cholesterol:* 0mg, *Fiber:* 1g, *Protein:* 8g, *Carbohydrate:* 43g, *Sugar:* 19g, *Sodium:* 55mg

SUPER NUTRIENTS
Vitamin A: 70%, Vitamin C: 212%, Vitamin K: 765%, Copper: 231%, Potassium: 1124mg

Extreme Green

This fruit-free green infusion is not for the faint of heart. Enjoy this cancer-fighting, chlorophyll-rich juice with a dash of chlorella and really take it to the next level!

INGREDIENTS
½ head romaine lettuce
3 celery stalks
1 handful cilantro
5–6 kale leaves
½ cucumber
1 handful spinach
¼ teaspoon chlorella (optional)

Juice all ingredients except the chlorella. Mix in chlorella, if desired.

NUTRITIONAL INFORMATION
Calories: 144, *Fat:* 3g, *Saturated Fat:* 0g, *Cholesterol:* 0mg, *Fiber:* 1g, *Protein:* 15g, *Carbohydrate:* 24g, *Sugar:* 5g, *Sodium:* 120mg

SUPER NUTRIENTS
Vitamin A: 296%, *Vitamin C:* 192%, *Vitamin K:* 1062%, Copper: 230%, Folate: 101%, Iron: 136%

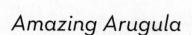

Amazing Arugula

Arugula is known for its anti-cancer effects, and cilantro is an amazing detoxifier. Together they make a very bold juice! I like to spike this juice with a bit of coconut water to even out the flavors.

INGREDIENTS
5 stalks celery
1 handful arugula
1 handful spinach
1 handful cilantro
1 apple, cored

Juice.

NUTRITIONAL INFORMATION
Calories: 58, *Fat:* 1g, *Saturated Fat:* 0g, *Cholesterol:* 0mg, *Fiber:* 1g, *Protein:* 2g, *Carbohydrate:* 18g, *Sugar:* 12g, *Sodium:* 75mg

SUPER NUTRIENT
Vitamin K: 155%

Broccomania

This green juice is chock-full of immune-boosting vitamin C and cancer-fighting sulforaphane!

INGREDIENTS
1 cucumber
1 small head broccoli
1 handful mint
1 lemon
1 apple, cored

Juice.

NUTRITIONAL INFORMATION
Calories: 186, Fat: 2g, Saturated Fat: 0g, Cholesterol: 0mg, Fiber: 2g, Protein: 14g, Carbohydrate: 54g, Sugar: 23g, Sodium: 147mg

SUPER NUTRIENTS
Vitamin C: 458%, Vitamin K: 391%, Iron: 51%

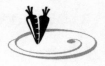

metric conversions

The recipes in this book have not been tested with metric measurements, so some variations might occur.

Remember that the weight of dry ingredients varies according to the volume or density factor: 1 cup of flour weighs far less than 1 cup of sugar, and 1 tablespoon doesn't necessarily hold 3 teaspoons.

GENERAL FORMULA FOR METRIC CONVERSION

Ounces to grams	multiply ounces by 28.35
Grams to ounces	multiply ounces by 0.035
Pounds to grams	multiply pounds by 453.5
Pounds to kilograms	multiply pounds by 0.45
Cups to liters	multiply cups by 0.24
Fahrenheit to Celsius	subtract 32 from Fahrenheit temperature, multiply by 5, divide by 9
Celsius to Fahrenheit	multiply Celsius temperature by 9, divide by 5, add 32

VOLUME (LIQUID) MEASUREMENTS

1 teaspoon = 1/6 fluid ounce = 5 milliliters

1 tablespoon = ½ fluid ounce = 15 milliliters

2 tablespoons = 1 fluid ounce = 30 milliliters

¼ cup = 2 fluid ounces = 60 milliliters

⅓ cup = 2 ⅔ fluid ounces = 79 milliliters

½ cup = 4 fluid ounces = 118 milliliters

1 cup or ½ pint = 8 fluid ounces = 250 milliliters

2 cups or 1 pint = 16 fluid ounces = 500 milliliters

4 cups or 1 quart = 32 fluid ounces = 1,000 milliliters

1 gallon = 4 liters

VOLUME (DRY) MEASUREMENTS

¼ teaspoon = 1 milliliter

½ teaspoon = 2 milliliters

¾ teaspoon = 4 milliliters

1 teaspoon = 5 milliliters

1 tablespoon = 15 milliliters

¼ cup = 59 milliliters

⅓ cup = 79 milliliters

½ cup = 118 milliliters

⅔ cup = 158 milliliters

¾ cup = 177 milliliters

1 cup = 225 milliliters

4 cups or 1 quart = 1 liter

½ gallon = 2 liters

1 gallon = 4 liters

WEIGHT (MASS) MEASUREMENTS

1 ounce = 30 grams
   2 ounces = 55 grams

3 ounces = 85 grams

4 ounces = ¼ pound = 125 grams

8 ounces = ½ pound = 240 grams

12 ounces = ¾ pound = 375 grams

16 ounces = 1 pound = 454 grams

LINEAR MEASUREMENTS

½ in = 1 ½ cm

1 inch = 2 ½ cm

6 inches = 15 cm

8 inches = 20 cm

10 inches = 25 cm

12 inches = 30 cm

20 inches = 50 cm

OVEN TEMPERATURE EQUIVALENTS, FAHRENHEIT (F) AND CELSIUS (C)

100°F = 38°C

....

200°F = 95°C

....

250°F = 120°C

....

300°F = 150°C

....

350°F = 180°C

....

400°F = 205°C

....

450°F = 230° C

....

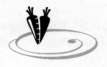

fruit and vegetable
nutrient table

Is your diet a little low in calcium? Need to boost your folic acid intake? How about more vitamin C? I love being able to customize my juice to target specific nutrients. Use the following table to create your own nutrient-rich cocktail by combining targeted fruits and vegetables together.

NUTRIENT YOU WANT	HOW TO GET IT
Calcium	Arugula, broccoli, celery, collards, garlic, kale, oranges, parsley, spinach
Choline	Greens, broccoli, cabbage, cauliflower
Chromium	Broccoli, garlic, romaine, spinach, tomatoes, wheatgrass
Coenzyme Q10	Broccoli, cabbage, spinach
Folic acid	Arugula, beets, bell peppers, cabbage, cauliflower, collards, dark leafy greens, lettuce, oranges, parsley, parsnips, spinach, sprouts, wheatgrass
Iodine	Cabbage, cucumbers, garlic, dark leafy greens, squash
Iron	Sprouts, beets, cabbage, dark leafy greens, lettuce, kale, mint, parsley, spinach, wheatgrass
Magnesium	Sprouts, dark greens, broccoli, cabbage, celery, garlic, ginger, parsley, parsnip, wheatgrass
Manganese	Apples, beets, carrots, cabbage, celery, kale, parsley, sweet potatoes, wheatgrass
Molybdenum	Carrots, cauliflower, sprouts, dark greens
Phosphorus	Broccoli, cabbage, cauliflower, dark leafy greens, leeks, parsley, parsnips, sweet potatoes, wheatgrass
Potassium	Greens, sprouts, and most other veggies!

Selenium	Asparagus, broccoli, Brussels sprouts, garlic, onions, sprouts
Sodium	Sprouts, beets, carrots, celery, dark leafy greens
Vitamin A (beta-carotene)	Greens, sprouts, beets, bell peppers, broccoli, cabbage, carrots, celery, chard, collards, dark leafy greens, fennel, lettuce, kale, parsley, squash, sweet potatoes, tomatoes, watermelon
B vitamins	Asparagus, beets, bok choy, broccoli, Brussels sprouts, cabbage, carrots, cauliflower, celery, cucumber, fennel, lemon, lime, oranges, parsnip, sprouts, watermelon, wheatgrass
Vitamin C	Bell peppers, broccoli, cabbage, cantaloupe, carrots, cauliflower, celery, collards, dark leafy greens, fennel, grapefruit, lemon, lime, oranges, parsley, parsnip, sprouts, tomatoes, sweet potatoes, watermelon, wheatgrass
Vitamin E	Asparagus, dark leafy greens, bell peppers, parsley, sprouts, watercress, wheatgrass
Vitamin K	Broccoli, cabbage, carrots, cauliflower, celery, cucumber, dark leafy greens, parsley, sprouts, wheatgrass
Vitamin D	Dark leafy greens, sprouts
Zinc	Broccoli, dark leafy greens, fennel, parsley, spinach, squash, sprouts, wheatgrass

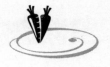

resources

On the following pages are the brands that I recommend to make juicing and living a detox lifestyle easy. Many of the superfoods can be found at your local grocery store as well as the websites provided.

SUPERFOOD	WEBSITE
Aloe vera	Lilyofthedesert.com
Chlorella	Chlorellafactor.com
	Sourcenaturals.com
	Sunchlorella.com
Cacao nibs	Navitas.com
	Sunfood.com
	Terramazon.com
Cereal Swag	Foodconfidence.com
Chia seeds	Navitas.com
	Salbasmart.com
	Spectrum.com
	Sunwarrior.com
	Truroots.com
Coconut oil	Artisana.com
	Kelapo.com
Coconut water	Harmlessharvest.com
Dandy Blend	Amazon.com
Flax seeds	Arrowheadmills.com
	Barleans.com
	Bobsredmill.com
	Carringtonfarms.com
	Spectrum.com
Hemp hearts	Manitobaharvest.com

Kelp powder	Nuts.com
	Seaveg.com
	Starwest-botanicals.com
Matcha tea powder	Domatcha.com
	Matchadna.com
Reishi mushroom extract	Dragonherbs.com
Sprouts	Sproutpeople.org
Salad Swag	Foodconfidence.com
Smoothie Swag	Foodconfidence.com
Spirulina	Nutrex-hawaii.com
Teechino	Teechino.com
Wheatgrass	Sproutpeople.org

TOOLS AND APPLIANCES	WEBSITE
Juicers	Breville.com
	Hurom.com
	Lexenjuicer.info/lexenmanual. html
	Omegajuicers.com
	Powerjuicer.com
	Samsonjuicers.com
High-speed blenders	Blendtec.com
	Ninjakitchen.com
	Nutribullet.com
	Vitamix.com

Ball Mason jars and lids	Amazon.com Cuppow.com
Evert Green Bags	Evertfresh.com
Knives	Crateandbarrel.com Target.com Williamssonoma.com
Dry skin brush	Amazon.com Target.com Yerba.com
Supplements	
Probiotics	Culterelle.com Florastor.com Rephreshprob.com Ultimateflora.com VSL3.com
Fish oil/omega-3 fats	Barleans.com Carlsons.com Nordicnaturals.com
Vitamin D	Carlsons.com Naturemade.com Nordicnaturals.com

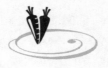

notes

1. Sonia F. Shenoy et al., "The Use of a Commercial Vegetable Juice as a Practical Means to Increase Vegetable Intake: A Randomized Controlled Trial," *Nutrition Journal* 9:38 (17 September 2010), DOI: 10.1186/1475-2891-9-38.

2. Sonia F. Shenoy et al., "Weight Loss in Individuals with Metabolic Syndrome Given DASH Diet Counseling When Provided a Low Sodium Vegetable Juice: A Randomized Controlled Trial," *Nutrition Journal* 9:8 (23 February 2010), DOI: 10.1186/1475-2891-9-8.

3. Dianne Hyson, Deborah Studebaker-Hallman, Paula A. Davis, and M. Eric Gershwin, "Apple Juice Consumption Reduces Plasma Low-Density Lipoprotein Oxidation in Healthy Men and Women," *Journal of Medicinal Food* 3, no. 4 (Winter 2000), DOI: 10.1089/jmf.2000.3.159.

4. S. Y. Kim, S. Yoon, S. M. Kwon, K. S. Park, and Y. C. Lee-Kim, "Kale Juice Improves Coronary Artery Disease Risk Factors in Hypercholesterolemic Men," *Journal of Biomedical and Environmental Sciences* 21, no. 2 (April 2008), DOI: 10.1016/S0895-3988(08)60012-4.

5. A. S. Potter, S. Foroudi, A. Stamatikos, B. S. Patil, and F. Deyhim, "Drinking Carrot Juice Increases Total Antioxidant Status and Decreases Lipid Peroxidation in Adults," *Nutrition Journal* 10:96 (24 September 2011), DOI: 10.1186/1475-2891-10-96.

6. Q. Dai, A. R. Borenstein, Y. Wu, J. C. Jackson, and E. B. Larson, "Fruit and Vegetable Juices and Alzheimer's Disease: The Kame Project," *American Journal of Medicine* 119, no. 9 (September 2006).

7. C. Morand et al., "Hesperidin Contributes to the Vascular Protective Effects of Orange Juice: A Randomized Crossover Study in Healthy Volunteers," *American Journal of Clinical Nutrition* 93 (January 2011), DOI: 10.3945/ajcn.110.004945.

8. Carrie H. S. Ruxto, Elaine J. Gardner, and Drew Walker, "Can Pure Fruit and Vegetable Juices Protect Against Cancer and Cardiovascular Disease Too? A Review of the Evidence," *International Journal of Food Sciences and Nutrition* 57, no. 3–4 (2006), DOI:10.1080/09637480600858134.

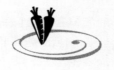

bibliography

"Bisphenol A (BPA)." http://www.niehs.nih.gov/health/assets/
docs_a_e/bisphenol-a-factsheet.pdf

"Bisphenol A (BPA): Expanding Research to Impact Human
Health National Institute of Environmental Health Sciences
(NIH)." http://www.niehs.nih.gov/research/supported/recovery/
critical/bpa/index.cfm

"Bisphenol A Fact Sheet National Toxicology Program." http://
www.who.int/mediacentre/factsheets/fs225/en/

Calafat, A. M., X. Ye, L. Y. Wong, J. A. Reidy, and L.L. Needham.
"Exposure of the US Population to Bisphenol A and 4-tertiary-
octylphenol: 2003–2004." *Environmental Health Perspectives*
(March 2004).

Dai, Q., A. R. Borenstein, Y. Wu, J. C. Jackson, and E. B. Larson. "Fruit and Vegetable Juices and Alzheimer's Disease: The Kame Project." *American Journal of Medicine* 119, no. 9 (September 2006).

"Dioxins and Their Effects on Human Health." http://www.who. int/mediacentre/factsheets/fs225/en/

Hayes, T. B., et al. "Atrazine Induces Complete Feminization and Chemical Castration in Male African Clawed Frogs (*Xenopus laevis*)." *Proceedings of the National Academy of Sciences* 107, no. 10 (March 9, 2010).

Hyman, Dr. Mark. *The Blood Sugar Solution*. New York: Little, Brown, 2012.

Hyson, Dianne, Deborah Studebaker-Hallman, Paula A. Davis, and M. Eric Gershwin. "Apple Juice Consumption Reduces Plasma Low-Density Lipoprotein Oxidation in Healthy Men and Women." *Journal of Medicinal Food* 3, no. 4 (Winter 2000). DOI: 10.1089/jmf.2000.3.159.

Kim, S. Y., S. Yoon, S. M. Kwon, K. S. Park, and Y. C. Lee-Kim, "Kale Juice Improves Coronary Artery Disease Risk Factors in Hypercholesterolemic Men." *Journal of Biomedical and Environmental Sciences* 21, no. 2 (April 2008). DOI: 10.1016/ S0895–3988(08)60012–4.

Morand, C., et al., "Hesperidin Contributes to the Vascular Protective Effects of Orange Juice: A Randomized Crossover

Study in Healthy Volunteers." *American Journal of Clinical Nutrition* 93 (January 2011). DOI: 10.3945/ajcn.110.004945.

Potter, A. S., S. Foroudi, A. Stamatikos, B. S. Patil, and F. Deyhim. "Drinking Carrot Juice Increases Total Antioxidant Status and Decreases Lipid Peroxidation in Adults." *Nutrition Journal* 10:96 (24 September 2011). DOI: 10.1186/1475–2891–10–96.

"PVC and Phthalates." http://www.noharm.org/us_canada/issues/toxins/pvc_phthalates/resources.php

Ruxto, Carrie H. S., Elaine J. Gardner, and Drew Walker. "Can Pure Fruit and Vegetable Juices Protect Against Cancer and Cardiovascular Disease Too? A Review of the Evidence." *International Journal of Food Sciences and Nutrition* 57, no. 3–4 (2006). DOI:10.1080/09637480600858134.

Samsel, A., and S. Seneff. "Glyphosate's Suppression of Cytochrome P450 Enzymes and Amino Acid Biosynthesis by the Gut Microbiome: Pathways to Modern Diseases." *Entropy* 15, no. 4 (2013).

Shenoy, Sonia F., et al. "The Use of a Commercial Vegetable Juice as a Practical Means to Increase Vegetable Intake: A Randomized Controlled Trial." *Nutrition Journal* 9, no. 38 (17 September 2010). DOI: 10.1186/1475–2891–9-38.

Shenoy, Sonia F., et al. "Weight Loss in Individuals with Metabolic Syndrome Given DASH Diet Counseling When

Provided a Low Sodium Vegetable Juice: A Randomized Controlled Trial." Nutrition Journal 9:8 (23 February 2010). DOI: 10.1186/1475-2891-9-8.

Suzawa, M., and H. A. Ingraham. "The Herbicide Atrazine Activates Endocrine Gene Networks via Non-Steroidal NR5A Nuclear Receptors in Fish and Mammalian Cells." *PLOS ONE* 3, no. 5 (2008).

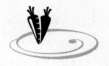

acknowledgments

I would like to thank the following people for their support, advice, and dedication to me, my vision, and the completion of this book.

To Holly and Renee: thanks to you both for this amazing opportunity and for giving me a chance.

To Hany and Norah: thank you for putting up with copious amounts of fresh produce in the fridge and the long days at my computer, and for being my two biggest fans.

To my clients and detoxers: thank you for being my inspiration and truly the reason I wrote this book. You have taught me so much over the years and I am grateful and honored to work with each and every one of you.

To my partner-in-kitchen, Ryan: thank you for your support, patience, wisdom, and encouragement during this entire project, and for always saying yes to the question, "Do you think this would taste good?" And also to my assistant, Nicole, thank you for your perseverance and dedication to the nutrition analysis. You were truly a life saver!

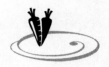

index

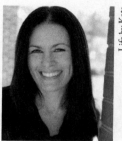

DANIELLE OMAR is a registered dietitian, culinary nutritionist, and healthy living expert. She has helped thousands of people achieve food confidence through teaching, speaking, and writing. Visit her online at www.foodconfidence.com.